THE
BOXER'S
CORNER

THE
BOXER'S
CORNER

*A Cancer Caregiver's Story
of Love, Loss, and Isolation*

MIGUEL BARRON

LIL'EG
PUBLISHING

Published by Lil'Eg Publishing,
Rancho Palos Verdes, California
www.theboxerscorner.com

Edited and designed by Girl Friday Productions
www.girlfridayproductions.com

Design: Paul Barrett
Project management: Sara Addicott
Image credits: Cover photo by Inked Pixels / Shutterstock;
All interior photos courtesy of Miguel Barron

ISBN (paperback): 978-1-7336228-0-6
ISBN (ebook): 978-1-7336228-1-3
LCCN: 2019905063

First edition

To Ivan and Luca, the joys of Nadia's life.

PREFACE

The idea of writing this book came to me about a year and a half into my wife's battle with breast cancer. Her initial diagnosis, in May 2013, set in motion the medical nightmare so many unfortunate women have to endure: a mastectomy, an axillary dissection, chemotherapy, and radiation treatment. By December of that year, seven long months after her initial diagnosis, her treatments finally appeared to be behind her.

Little did we know that only a few short months after finishing her array of treatments, a dry and persistent cough would reveal her cancer had returned, this time to her lungs.

What my wife and so many other women have battled is nothing less than brutal: the physical abuse of surgery after surgery, the agonizing marathon that is chemotherapy, and the psychological distress of losing one's "femininity"—breast loss, hair loss, weight volatility, and skin changes. As if that weren't enough, there is the small matter of *the fear of death*. More specifically, the fear of dying at a young age, of leaving everything one loves behind, one's children, one's husband, one's friends, everything.

I can never pretend to understand how lonely my wife must have felt at times. But I have a very good idea of how much she suffered. And I do because I have witnessed all of it in person from the very first minute. In doing so, I have experienced profound pain and loneliness myself. And that is what prompted me to write these pages.

I know I am not the victim here. Few things can compare with the mental and physical suffering of a woman's fight with breast cancer. But while the world is well designed to provide support to cancer patients—through family, friends, doctors, counselors, and, of course, the spouse, I found few obvious outlets for the emotional roller coaster I was facing.

Writing these pages became my way of coping. It helped me digest and come to terms with all the emotions I was feeling. And it spared my friends the extra hours (and there were plenty) of hearing about my wife's seemingly endless struggle. I also wanted to leave a transcript of events for my sons,

Ivan and Luca, who were too young to compre-
hend everything that was happening, but who may
one day read these pages and better understand
what happened to their mother. And should these
pages ever reach other caregivers fighting to save a
loved one, I hope those readers find some solace in
knowing they are not alone and that it is okay to be
overwhelmed by the responsibilities and pressure
involved with being "the strong one." That many of
the conflicting emotions they may be experiencing
are natural. That many of the frustrations they feel
are nothing to be ashamed of.

I am not a doctor or psychologist. I cannot speak
in scientific terms about how one may or should
feel. I can only provide my own personal experience as a reference. And should these pages ever
reach others in similar circumstances, I hope they
serve as a source of solidarity and companionship.

And to my wonderful Ivan and Luca, this was
the story of your father's battle to save your beautiful mother.

Ignorance Is Bliss

It was a perfectly normal weeknight, maybe a
Tuesday or a Wednesday. We had recently returned

from a ski trip out West and were slowly getting back into our daily routine. The boys were upstairs getting ready for bed, and I was lying in bed watching TV while Nadia changed in the bathroom. It was as normal a night as any. While she stood in front of the mirror, I noticed Nadia holding up her left arm. She seemed to repeat a motion with her arm, raising it and then lowering it, while periodically feeling her left breast with the fingers of her right hand. I didn't really pay attention to it and would have never remembered, if not for what ultimately transpired. Nonchalantly, she turned her head toward me and said, "I think I feel a little something here."

I walked into the bathroom and placed my finger on the exact location she was indicating. "I don't really feel anything," I replied. "But make an appointment with the doctor if you want." The truth is that I did not really feel anything. And yet, I had a strange, uneasy feeling about it, which I knew made little sense from any rational standpoint. But without fretting on it any further, we agreed she would make an appointment with her doctor the next day and left it at that.

It took some two to three weeks before Nadia saw her doctor, possibly due to the doctor's busy schedule or Nadia's putting off making the appointment for a few days. In any case, by the time she went to see her doctor, the "little something" was very much noticeable. I could now roll my finger over it, as if it were a small marble deep under her skin. The doctor eventually saw her and, as was to be expected, requested a biopsy of the "little something" in her breast.

In the days following the biopsy, Nadia became increasingly nervous. She knew breast cancer was very common, and there seemed to be little other explanation for why there would be a small lump in her breast. I tried to comfort her by telling her it was probably nothing, a cyst or something of the sort. And so the days passed while we waited to hear from the doctor.

One day after work, while I was having drinks with colleagues, my phone rang. I had warned Nadia I would be running late, and she was well accustomed to the "lads'" post-work drinks ritual. So there was no real reason to call me, other than, of course, to tell me she had news of the lab results. Before I picked up the phone, I knew what the call was about. And just as I had feared, the voice on the other end was that of my frightened wife, crying.

"It's cancer, Papa. It's cancer." The dreaded words that would forever change our lives.

From the moment of my wife's initial diagnosis, I was hell-bent on learning everything I could about breast cancer in general and about *her* breast cancer in particular. I discovered very quickly that speaking about breast cancer in generic terms is a bit like speaking about cars in generic terms. We know cars have wheels and brakes and lights, but a Lamborghini has little in common with a Toyota. Overall, breast-cancer statistics are very encouraging, and they get better every year. But when you peel that onion, you discover there are huge differences in the risk profiles of different subtypes—something I would have never known had I not been plunged into the matter headfirst.

When I was handed a copy of my wife's first biopsy report—the one of the original tumor—it was like looking at a Chinese manuscript. I didn't understand a word. What I did notice, however, was that Nadia's doctor and her assistant had managed to shuffle all of their meetings around in order to block out a full hour of their day to discuss the test results with us.

The clinic was conveniently located in our town, and we had made an early-morning appointment. It was a weekday and there were few people around, which helped ease our anxiety. We were called into the doctor's office, and we waited nervously in the quiet and sparsely furnished room. When the doctor and assistant walked in, they were professional, deliberate, and warm. But I was feeling uneasy about how hard they were trying to be calm. As I would later learn, physicians (and especially oncologists) are well trained in the art of communication management. Many months and dozens of consultations later, I could practically tell you what they were going to say in advance. More importantly, I could tell you what they *weren't* going to say.

But back to the biopsy report and the doctor. Despite reassuring us that everything would be fine and that breast-cancer treatment had made great strides in recent years, they did eventually come clean and acknowledge that my wife's cancer was "a little on the aggressive side." I, of course, had no idea what that meant. So I did what any concerned spouse would do. I spent the next seventy-two hours poring over the pathology report, trying to make sense of it.

As it turns out, and without dwelling too much on the technical, there are certain tests in a tumor biopsy that are designed to measure the aggressiveness of a cancer: mitosis count, nuclear count, and tubule formation. These are sometimes added together to produce a "score" in something called the Nottingham Grade. The best score—the least aggressive one—is a 3 (1+1+1). The worst is a 9 (3+3+3). On the Nottingham Grade, Nadia's score was an 8, which was later revised to 9 upon completion of the full lab work. Her tumor cells were "poorly differentiated," meaning they did not look very similar to regular cells, usually a sign of more aggressive cancers. Other important prognostic factors were also working against her. For starters, her age. The average age of a breast-cancer patient in the US is fifty-four and a half. Nadia was forty-two at initial diagnosis. It is well documented that cancer tends to be more aggressive among younger patients. Other indicators such as her tumor size (3.2 cm) and proliferation rate (Ki-67 > 15%) also fell on the risky side. But the two biggest red flags were yet to come.

Given the risk profile of Nadia's breast cancer, it was clear she would require a mastectomy, which we promptly scheduled. During the course of a mastectomy (the removal of the breast), it is common for the surgeon to remove a few lymph nodes to see if the cancer has spread into the lymphatic system. Cancer can spread through the bloodstream or through the lymphatic system. So finding cancerous lymph nodes is a pretty big deal. It means that at least from a local-regional standpoint, the cat is out of the bag. Given how aggressive Nadia's cancer type was, we definitely wanted it to be contained. Unfortunately we were not so lucky. Of the three nodes removed during the procedure, two tested positive. This meant that after she recovered from the mastectomy, she would have to schedule an axillary dissection—an operation to remove more lymph nodes in order to see how many more were cancerous. In Nadia's case, they took out another seventeen nodes and found an additional three that were positive. Her subsequent pathology report cited "extensive lympho-vascular invasion," corroborating that the cancer had not been contained in the breast.

The second red flag had to do with the all-important hormone receptors. When a tumor is removed and its tissue sent to the lab, it is tested for hormone receptors. Breast-cancer cells are typically *fueled* by one of three hormones: ER (estrogen), PR (progesterone), or the epidermal growth-factor receptor HER2. If tumors are "expressing" for one of these, then chemotherapy will typically be accompanied or followed by a targeted hormone treatment to deprive or neutralize the cancer of its *energy* source. Cancers that can be targeted usually have a better prognosis, as they are more likely to respond to treatment. And some of the greatest cancer breakthroughs in recent years have occurred in this fast-developing field called immuno-oncology. If, however, the tumors are not express-ing for any of the three hormones, they are referred to as *triple-negative* breast cancers. These represent only between 15 to 20 percent of all breast-cancer cases, but they are very difficult to treat and have worse overall prognoses. Once again, we man-aged to draw the worst card in the deck. Her lab work (using a method called IHC—immunohisto-chemistry) showed that her tumors were not expressing for *any* of the three hormones. *So we were stuck with an aggressive cancer that had left the scene of the crime (spread to the lymph nodes) and was going to be hard to treat (triple negative).*

Adding it all up, it wasn't hard to come to the conclusion that Nadia's risk of cancer recurrence was high. None of the doctors were ever going to be that explicit, but it was clear from the various data points I was collecting that her subtype was not an easy one. I also knew that if her cancer ever did return (to a distant organ—bones, lungs, liver, or brain), she would technically be a stage IV cancer patient. At that point the disease would be treatable but no longer curable. In other words, *if her cancer ever returned, her condition would be terminal.*

Of course, Nadia wasn't doing any of this type of research. She was scared enough as it was and overwhelmed by the physical demands of surgeries and treatments. Nadia preferred to listen to her doctors and hold on to every hopeful word that came out of their mouths. She didn't really want to know about the deep, dark details of her disease. This was her way of coping. It was also what the doctors recommended, and what I constantly reinforced. "Don't read the internet. It will drive you nuts and scare you unnecessarily. Those statistics are deceiving. Everybody is different. Just be positive."

I played into that rhetoric daily. I knew that it was my responsibility to keep her thinking positively. If there was ever bad news to be dispensed, it would be the responsibility of the doctors, not me, to disseminate it. And so week after week, month after month, I perfected my cheerleading skills, all the while knowing privately that her particular prognosis was a dangerous one.

There is a prognostic calculator called NPI (Nottingham Prognostic Index), which is used to assess a breast-cancer patient's overall risk. There is nothing magical about it, and it is by no means a Holy Grail in its predictive qualities. But it can be used to put a patient into one of four prognosis

groups: excellent, good, moderate, or poor. Taking
the tumor size, the histological grade, and the
number of positive lymph nodes, a formula is run:
$(0.2 \times S) + N + G$. The resulting score—the NPI—
places patients into one of the following prognostic
categories:

Excellent: 2–2.4
Good: > 2.4–3.4
Moderate: > 3.4–4.4
Poor: > 4.4–5.4

Nadia scored a 6.6, putting her pretty much
off the charts. Again, I learned all of this through
research of my own. *And as I would learn, these
were not the kind of data points doctors willingly
volunteer.*

As I continued reading and learning about the
disease, I would occasionally disclose my findings
to very close friends in confidence. But I would
never tell Nadia about it. And she would never discover it on her own. *She made sure she didn't.*

All the while, we kept meeting with our oncologist before every round of chemo. I started observ-
ing the carefully chosen words and phrases she
used. She would always be *technically* correct, but
she would always mask the bigger picture. She knew

this was a tricky cancer but was never going to say it in as many words. As I would come to learn, the job of an oncologist is not just to administer chemo, but also to keep the patient in a positive state of mind. To this day I think our oncologist knew *that I knew* how aggressive Nadia's cancer was, but she avoided ever "going there." I could sometimes sense she would have preferred me not to be in the room when she met with Nadia. *My presence made the story harder to spin.*

Of Hunches and Lies

Not telling the whole truth about something for an extended period of time can be exhausting. When asked point-blank, "I'm going to be fine, right?" my answer always had to be, "Of course, my love." When the children asked me straight up, "Papa, Mama is going to be cured, right?" there was only one right answer, and that answer was only partially true: "Boys, she is in the very best hands and she is young and strong. There is no reason to be scared."

I needed to keep them hopeful and positive, but I didn't want to promise something I couldn't deliver. I needed to choose my words carefully. *I*

was playing the same game our oncologist was play-
ing with us, except I was doing it with my own wife
and children.

With the passage of time this really began to
wear on me. Lies are easy to deal with when they
die in the distant past. They are harder to handle
when you're muscled into telling them over and
over, every day. This is not to say that Nadia's des-
tiny was systematically doomed or predetermined.
There was a very decent chance (at least from my
research) that she would be cured and never deal
with cancer again. *But somehow I never had that*
feeling.

This is one of the things I struggled most with
during the course of her disease. From the very
first moment she stood in front of the bathroom
mirror and said, completely casually, "I think I feel
a little thing in my boob," I had a bad feeling. I have
mentioned this to close friends in the past, who I'm
sure thought I was being mystical or dramatic. But
it was true. And it was difficult to describe. I'm a
rational person who believes in math and science
and doesn't subscribe to tales of telepathy or ESP.
But sometimes you just have a feeling about something, for no reason whatsoever. Like when you're
watching a sporting event on TV and you are absolutely convinced something is going to happen,

and it does. It was silly and irrational, but I couldn't shake it.

As things turned out, my premonitions were correct. In the three weeks it took Nadia to go see a doctor about the little "thing" in her boob, the little pimple I couldn't even feel at first had grown to the size of a grape. By the day of her appointment, I could easily roll my finger over it. And every test and every lab report from that point on would do nothing but reinforce my fears—corroborate that *feeling.*

This made my role as "cheerleader of last resort" all the more difficult. I knew I was doing the right thing by staying positive and answering questions with a positive spin. But I felt like I was constantly *lying.* And to the few people I trusted enough to tell the truth, I would have to tamp down my concerns to accommodate their skepticism:

"Dude, these lab reports are horrible. I have a really bad feeling about this."

"C'mon, Mig. Don't be silly. She will be fine."

"Yeah, I guess you're probably right."

Of course, I didn't believe that. I had a very bad feeling about the whole thing, and every incremental piece of information I uncovered seemed to substantiate it. But I didn't want to come across as irrational or paranoid. This all made me feel extremely isolated. I felt like I was keeping a secret. Everybody around me *needed* to hear something other than what I really believed.

Au Revoir le Français

Nadia and I met in 1994 in Abu Dhabi. I was an analyst at ADIA, the sovereign wealth fund of Abu Dhabi, and Nadia had just returned to the Emirates to visit her mother and uncles after graduating from college in Pennsylvania. I was in no particular mood to fall in love. I had spent the prior two years chasing any young, unsuspecting expat girl who crossed my path. I was in my twenties, had a beautiful apartment, a nice car, and a couple of bucks to spend. Why would I ever complicate my life with anything deep, when the shallow end of the pool was perfectly fine?

As it turns out, that's not how life works. Love, as they say, has a mind of its own. I met Nadia on a night out with a friend. She had started dating a young Frenchman whose father ran the local operations of a major European oil company. As luck would have it, the young man went back to France on holiday for a few weeks in the summer. It was the perfect window of opportunity.

Nadia and I started to see each other quite a bit, sometimes with a group of friends and sometimes on our own. But I was falling for her fast. She was tall and thin, with long black hair, a beautiful smile, and big expressive eyes. She was Pakistani, although her family was originally from Bangladesh and had to move to West Pakistan after Bangladesh became independent. She was well educated and well traveled.

Despite our very different geographic and cultural backgrounds (my parents were both Spanish, and I grew up between California and Spain), we shared a similar outlook on life. We both valued our families and roots, but we both had a healthy disdain for the provincial or pedantic. We were both highly tolerant of other cultures and beliefs, and we were cynical of anybody who thought they had the world figured out. We were both privately spiritual, but both rejected the fanfare of institutionalized religion. But what I most appreciated about Nadia—in addition to her looks, of course— was her ability to laugh. Not just at anyone or anything, but mostly at herself. There was no situation she couldn't mock. I remember one morning, at the height of my libido, when I insisted we do it one more time. She sighed, rolled her eyes, and said, "Okay, just hand me that magazine."

We married a whole *six months* after meeting. It was crazy, but neither of us really cared. We didn't pay much attention to rules or what other people thought. Nobody was going to tell us what to do. And I wasn't about to lose the woman of my life to anybody else's opinion. So on March 19, 1995, we married in Dubai.

Our travels would later take us to London (briefly) and eventually to New York. We moved around a couple of more times during the course of the next twenty years, including three years in Madrid (from 2002 to 2005) and three in Miami (from 2005 to 2008). Our older son, Ivan, was born in New York; our younger son, Luca, in Madrid.

As the years went by, and we dealt with the normal stresses of responsibility and marriage, we would, like any other couple, bump heads fairly frequently. Nadia was the most stubborn person in the world, *after me*. Our marital spats were something to behold. They were the loud, crazy kind. Neither of us was capable of the quiet, stoic, Anglo-Saxon model of fighting. We subscribed to the vocal "in your face" method of dealing with our problems. Ironically, we agreed that our marriage lasted as long as it did because we didn't keep anything inside. If she was upset, it was the wrath of God (the expression "Hell hath no fury like a woman scorned" leaps to mind). Of course, my Spanish blood didn't make matters any easier. If I believed I was in the right, I couldn't back down. I called it "the 1 percent rule." I'm perfectly happy to let things go 99 percent of the time, but for that 1 percent, I'd burn the village before giving in. And so during the course of our marriage we learned that for the many periods of peace, there would be the occasional world war. But we learned to cope with it and respect each other all the more for it.

The One-Handed Fighter

Nadia's cancer changed all of that. The treatment she underwent was debilitating beyond what any of the doctors had warned. One lesson I took away from our experience was that doctors always seem to sugarcoat things. The mastectomy was supposed to be "no major deal." The hell it was. Nadia spent two nights at Weill Cornell barely able to move and vomiting nonstop in reaction to the anesthetic. The axillary dissection was supposed to be "pretty noninvasive and very much an outpatient type of procedure." Bullshit. She was in so much pain we had to wait until past midnight to move her anywhere. She suffered severe pain in both her arm and armpit for weeks afterward and had to go to rehabilitation to recover full movement in her arm. The chemo was also supposed to be "manageable." But it was much worse than either of us expected.

Managing all of these symptoms is a Pandora's box in itself. For every pain or ailment, there is a medication. And for each of the side effects of those medications, there is another medication. Nadia referred to it as the big Russian babushka doll. You keep peeling one off to find another smaller one inside, seemingly with no end. Her online patient portal with Weill Cornell and later Sloan Kettering listed all of the medications she had taken in addition to the chemo agents. The list went into the dozens.

It can be no surprise, then—given the physical and psychological trauma she had endured, and the plethora of medications she had ingested—that she would not be entirely herself. Nobody could possibly expect a person to behave normally under such circumstances. Unfortunately the patient doesn't always see that. Her mood swings were often wild and her behavior irrational. She could oscillate between deep depression and steroid-induced euphoria. She would experience fits of intense rage, often a product of going off a particular medication. And when those cycles hit, I was inevitably on the receiving end. I tried not to react, because I understood it wasn't really her. But she often needed her feelings validated and not dismissed as "medical." So you could never really *call it.* I tried, on a couple of occasions, to explain to her that she was just reacting to the meds and that it would pass. But those comments made matters worse. She was looking for validation, not a diagnosis—no matter how outrageous her reactions may have been.

And so, after years of standing up for myself and defending my corner, I found I could no longer do it. Like a one-handed fighter, I could duck and weave but I couldn't really throw a punch. There is no resentment in my saying this. I understood that none of this was her fault, and I know she didn't mean what she said or did on those occasions. But she would sometimes land pretty painful punches, all the same. *And when that happened, once again, the sense of isolation and loneliness would kick in.* I couldn't quite recognize the person yelling at me. I couldn't quite defend myself. And I couldn't really tell anyone about it. After all, I could never disrespect my wife enough to repeat in public some of the things she said to me. Similarly, I couldn't vent my frustration to a friend about my wife's crazy behavior. That, too, would be insensitive and disrespectful. *I never found a correct way of dealing with*

any of this. So with the passage of time, the pressure
kept building.

The Locker Room

All the while, I had a job to keep. And not your
typical nine-to-five job either. I was working on
the international equity-sales desk of a major Wall
Street investment bank (UBS). My day-to-day
began with an alarm clock going off at four a.m. I
would shower, get dressed, make coffee, and start
reading. First, I would cover the international business press (*Financial Times, Wall Street Journal,
Bloomberg*). Then, on the 5:09 train into Grand
Central, I would read our in-house research for
the day. By the time I got to the office around six,
I had a pretty good idea of what was going on in
the world. Except it wasn't really an office. It was a
large trading floor where we sat in long rows, each
person not more than two feet from another. This
was great for the purposes of the job. There was a
free flow of information and ideas that generated
a productive buzz. The format helped keep all of
us up to speed on what others were hearing and
doing, and it encouraged teamwork and communication. *Of course, if you were dealing with heavy*

personal issues or needed a little privacy, it was not the ideal setting.

During the course of my wife's multiple treatments and procedures, as well as the release of her many lab reports—biopsies, blood work, scans, and the like—I found it extremely difficult to keep my personal issues to myself while at work. You can try to put on a brave face and join in on the desk banter, but the closeness of it all made things difficult to hide. I had the good fortune of working with great friends and colleagues, who for the most part were much more the former than the latter. I was also fortunate to have a boss with a significant sense of humanity, a rare breed in today's financial world. But despite the leeway I was afforded, I always felt very conscious of how much my personal issues were filtering into my day-to-day at work. *It is very hard to hide your emotions when you spend twelve hours a day in what is essentially a high-tech locker room.*

If I had a bad night or was worried about a lab report or an upcoming procedure, I wore it on my face. Some people are very good at hiding their emotions. As much as I try, I'm just not one of them. This began to concern me greatly with the passing of every month. *Unlike other problems, cancer does not have a defined timeline.* I had no idea how long my wife would be sick. I had no idea how many more consultations or procedures lay ahead. I had no idea if, and when, her cancer would recur. And once it did, I had no idea how long she would be able to hold out, or what her condition would be during treatment. The situation became unmanageable for me and visibly noticeable to my colleagues.

Our line of work was particularly demanding. We were under constant stress, and anybody could get fired pretty much at any time. It was hard enough to do the job with all of your faculties in good working order. It was altogether impossible if you had the weight of the world on your shoulders.

The Sleeping Passenger

By December 2013, Nadia's plethora of treatments finally came to an end. She had endured countless visits to clinics and emergency rooms, a mastectomy, an axillary dissection, rounds of chemotherapy and radiation, rehabilitation treatment, and ingesting an endless list of unpronounceable medications. Our sense of relief was total and difficult to describe. Cancer treatment doesn't just require physical and psychological strain, it completely consumes your life. Your schedule is based entirely on preparing for, attending, or recovering from some type of medical-related issue or procedure. You cannot plan anything outside of those parameters. It dictates every aspect of your life. To look at a blank calendar again gave us a sense of freedom and respite we had thought would never return.

To celebrate the occasion, I organized a dinner at our favorite New York restaurant with a group of our close friends, who had been such a great source of love and support to us throughout Nadia's treatment. It was as much a celebration of the end of Nadia's treatment as it was a big "thank-you" to these great friends for all they had done for us. We had a multi-hour dinner, with plenty of wine, customized menus marking the occasion, and, more importantly, many much-needed laughs. We ended the night with emotional hugs and kisses, and Nadia went to bed that night believing her nightmare had ended and her life was back to normal.

I had participated in the celebration with a genuine sense of relief: The relief of knowing that I no longer had to witness my wife's suffering. The relief of knowing she would slowly regain strength, feel better, and become more active. The relief of knowing we could now plan activities as a family and that my children could enjoy their mother again.

But in the back of my mind, I knew it was not that simple. I knew that we now had a very different enemy to combat. Our adversary from that point on was silent and invisible. An intangible force that lulls you into complacency by its sheer absence of presence. It was the polar opposite of the noise and disruption of medical treatments, hospitals, and doctors. Our new enemy was *time*.

The risk of cancer recurrence can be statistically compartmentalized into years. The more time goes by without recurrence, the lower the probability of its return. The key hurdles are usually set at three, five, and ten years. Every day that passes without cancer recurrence increases your odds of overall survival (referred to as OAS in survival statistics). I knew that every uneventful day was a little step forward in saving her. Of course, Nadia didn't think along these lines. Nadia was convinced, or had managed to convince herself, that it was all over. She didn't understand terms like "disease-free progression" or "overall survival rate" and had no interest in learning about them.

And so, like a driver with a sleeping passenger, I would quietly celebrate the collisions we managed to avoid every day, while my fellow traveler enjoyed the journey in perfect bliss.

Unfortunately, closing your eyes doesn't mean something isn't there. The risk was real and ever present in my mind. I was trying to enjoy our new normal life, but a part of me was holding my breath. I constantly felt like a golfer who sprayed a tee shot out over a busy highway and was cringing, hoping to not hear a sound. Every day felt like another second without a sound—*phew, good news.* I repeated the act day after day, week after week, celebrating each one privately as a small victory.

And so we carried on for a few short, happy months. Until one day the silence finally broke, and the passenger was forced to wake from her peaceful sleep.

Mañana

Once my wife's cancer returned, the stakes changed. I had always feared it would—that *feeling*—but when a lady in a white coat says your wife can no longer be cured, it hits home hard.

We were vacationing at my parents' home in Marbella, in southern Spain, in summer, only a few months after Nadia had finished her treatments. Prior to our trip Nadia had developed a dry, nagging cough that strangely wasn't accompanied by any of the other symptoms one would expect—no fever, no phlegm, no runny nose. Nothing. As conscious as I was of the ever-present risk of recurrence, I really wouldn't have expected it to come back so soon. Could this really be the cancer again? I mean, how could it come back so quickly? If so, it would be as if *her first chemo regimen had done absolutely nothing to halt the progression of the disease.*

Once we were in Marbella, the cough got pretty bad. Despite our disagreement as to how long she had been suffering from it—Nadia insisting it was very recent and probably nothing to worry about (of course) and me telling her exactly how many weeks it had been—it was serious enough that we had to visit a local clinic.

I had trained myself to be on the lookout for any signs indicative of recurrence. I knew the symptoms for each of the possible landing areas (bone, brain, liver, and, of course, lungs). I had first noticed the cough around the middle of June. She also seemed to have less of an appetite and had lost a little weight. The fact that the cough persisted and seemed to be getting worse, not better, without any accompanying flu-like symptoms, had me worried.

The next two days were surreal. We called the main hospital in Marbella and managed to get an appointment for the following day. We were both nervous, and Nadia's initial denial reflex had evolved into genuine concern. She didn't understand the concept of cancer recurrence or its implications to the extent I did. But she knew her cough was not normal, and she was scared. Once at the clinic, we met with the head of Pulmonology. He was a soft-spoken, mild-mannered man who addressed us warmly and exuded a certain calmness. He asked a number of questions, and I provided a brief synopsis of Nadia's medical history. He suggested an X-ray to have a preliminary look at her lungs. The slides were produced within the hour, and we went back to the doctor's office to get his take.

In one of those moments that will stay with me forever, I watched the doctor hold the slide up against a light and, without speaking, make a subtle facial expression. It was the look of somebody who has seen something but is making an effort not to react to it. Like the look on someone's face if they see a spider on your shoulder. He didn't say a word, and yet somehow, he gave it away. Nadia noticed it as well and jumped: "What? What is it?"

Taking his cue from what appears to be a universal doctor code of conduct, he explained calmly that there was something a little cloudy toward the bottom of the lungs that he wanted to take a closer look at. It was probably nothing, maybe an infection of some sort, but he needed to have a closer look. *I am convinced to this day that he knew at that moment what it was he was seeing.* But sticking to script, he calmed us down and kept the positive spin going as long as possible. He suggested a more detailed look via a CT scan and promised he would call us as soon as he got the results.

That same evening, Nadia received *the* phone call. Her Spanish was pretty good, so she tried her best to carry on the conversation. At one point, however, the doctor seemed to be saying something she couldn't quite understand, so she handed me the phone. She was beginning to panic and looked at me fearfully as I addressed the doctor. He told me he needed to see us first thing in the morning to discuss the results of the scan. At this point Nadia could smell a rat and started yelling over me, "What is he saying?? What is it?? Is it the cancer?? Is it back??" I had to move to another room just to hear what the doctor was saying.

"Miguel, Miguel, can you hear me?" the doctor asked politely. "Miguel, she has metastasis in her lungs. It's everywhere. I need to see you both in person tomorrow without fail. *Mañana sin falta.*"

The moment I hung up the phone, I was under assault. The doctor said he wanted to speak to

Nadia in person. It wasn't my job to convey bad news to my wife. I was the cheerleader, remember? The last bastion of good news and hope. I couldn't possibly be the one to tell her. But there was no stopping this.

She was screaming at the top of her lungs, "What did he say? Tell me, what did he say?"

Her eyes were full of rage and fear. It was so primal. My sense of duty as *cheerleader* was quickly overrun by a sense of loyalty and empathy to my life partner, to the mother of my children. She was panicking and demanding to know what the doctor had said. How could I keep it from her? So I told her. I had to. *And once I did, everything changed.*

From the very beginning, Nadia had dealt with her condition with a strong and healthy sense of denial. She had convinced herself everything would be fine and focused only on whatever positive reinforcement she received from her doctors, her friends and family, and from me. She never read about survival rates. She never read her own pathology reports. She never knew the difference between triple negative and ER positive, or anything else, for that matter. Her defense mechanism was to block everything out. It was difficult to discuss the disease with her at all without being shut down immediately. But after the Marbella incident, she would no longer have that luxury. This was a ticking time bomb, and she would have to come to terms with her condition, whether she wanted to or not. But Nadia being Nadia, I knew it would be a slow and difficult road.

We arrived at the clinic first thing the next morning as instructed. The doctor ushered us into his office and pulled up the three-dimensional images of Nadia's lungs on his PC. *He was right. The tumors were everywhere.* It was plain to see, even to my untrained eyes. He gave us a copy of the CD-ROM to take back to our oncologist in New York and wished us well. As we walked out of his office, I noticed the doctor looking at us. The look on his face was a combination of incredulity and pity, like a jury looking at a man who has just been sentenced to death. I sensed as we left that he must have felt like the unluckiest doctor in the world that day, having to deliver dreadful news to a couple of tourists who randomly stumbled into his office on a bright summer's day.

Spin Doctors

When we returned to New York, we took the CD-ROM to our oncologist at Weill Cornell. Our doctor was an Asian American woman who had always treated us well, albeit in a somewhat cold and transactional way, considering our circumstances. From the moment Nadia had begun her treatment, I always wondered what would compel someone to become an oncologist. I understand they are in the business of saving lives. But there was always something a little macabre, in my opinion, about making a living by poisoning people to their near death. But personality issues aside, and with all due respect, this was a person Nadia and I had hoped to never have to see again. Sadly, fate did not grant us this wish. So we braved our way to Manhattan's Upper East Side and handed our oncologist the CD-ROM.

The doctor conducted a PET/CT scan of her own to corroborate the one from Spain. Despite the fact that only two weeks had passed since the Marbella scan, the new report not only confirmed the metastasis, citing "innumerable pulmonary nodules," but went on to highlight "significant interval progression in both size and number" relative to the one from Spain. *So in just two weeks, the tumors had already grown in size and number.* To make matters worse, the PET scan found foci in both the liver and bones, *"concerning for hepatic and osseous metastases."* In other words, the CT scan confirmed all of the existing tumors in her lungs, and the PET scan, which measures suspicious metabolic activity (a sort of leading indicator), identified "concerning" activity in her liver and bones. As I had feared all along, *this was no Toyota. We were dealing with a Lamborghini.*

The scan was followed by biopsies of two of the tumors in her lungs. As if things weren't complicated enough, one of them expressed very slightly for ER (a 25 percent stain, as they call it) and the other "overexpressed" for HER2, albeit only slightly (2.2, which is considered moderate). *So her tumors were a hodgepodge of cancer—sometimes appearing as triple negative, other times expressing slightly for ER, and other times expressing slightly for HER2— depending on where the samples were taken.* Most of the successful drugs in the cancer space are designed to target one of the three hormone receptors (ER, PR, or HER2). And there are good clinical trials targeting triple-negative breast cancers as well. But what do you do if you have a little of everything and not enough of any one thing? How do you target that? *I was no doctor, but I knew this wasn't going to be easy.*

One of my ongoing frustrations throughout my wife's treatment was the growing discrepancy between what I was learning about her condition and what the doctors were actually telling her. It was becoming clear that bad news was only to be dispensed when absolutely necessary. And even when it was offered, it was communicated gently enough that a patient with my wife's general aversion to reality would take a while to actually *get it*. When our oncologist explained that my wife's cancer had in fact metastasized to both lungs, Nadia's response was something to the effect of, "So what does that mean?" I knew exactly what it meant. But Nadia needed to be told more explicitly. It took a lot of circling around, but the doctor—eventually remarking on Nadia's inability or unwillingness to understand—finally made it clear.

"This basically means that your disease is no longer *curable*, but we can *treat it*."

Again, the roadblock. "Yes, Doctor, but what does that *mean*?"

"It means that unless you get in a car accident or something like that, you are probably going to die of this. And the median survival is around three years, although many people do a lot better."

The doctor finally managed to say what she had to say. But between her well-rehearsed pauses and Nadia's natural blocking reflex, it all took a lot longer than I thought was necessary.

Nadia's takeaway from that meeting was that she had *at least* three years—and that she could probably do a lot better than that. And while I wanted to share her positive attitude, I knew that for every patient who does better than the average, there will be another who does considerably worse. It was math, pure and simple.

This was not the only example of our doctors spinning things—not by far. When Nadia had her first operation (the original mastectomy), the surgeon's staff asked for my cell number so they could contact me when the surgery was over. When I received the phone call, it was from the surgeon herself.

"How did it go, Doctor?" I asked.

"It went really well. I didn't see anything suspicious," she replied.

And yet, I soon found out that two of the three lymph nodes they had removed turned out to be cancerous. The bluff got even better after the axillary dissection that followed. As I mentioned earlier, this procedure would uncover another *three* cancerous lymph nodes. When we met with the surgeon to hear the test results, her medical summary went something like this: "Yes, there were three more positive nodes, but it's fine. Your skin margins were okay."

How could she possibly suggest that clean skin margins (i.e., there was no cancer on the skin tissue around the breast) were more important than five cancerous lymph nodes! The number of positive nodes is widely recognized as a critical indicator of recurrence risk—infinitely more so than skin margins. So much so that it is categorized into three risk groups: those with zero positive nodes (obviously the safest), those who find one to three nodes, and the worst group, with four or more positive nodes. Nadia had *five*. But there was absolutely no emphasis on the cancerous lymph nodes, only the good skin margins. It seemed clear to me that the doctor was banking on Nadia not knowing the relative significance of each of these so she would walk away with a more positive message.

Guinea Pigs and Pharma Bros

In discussing various treatment options, now that Nadia's cancer had returned, and given her specific subtype, our oncologist spent considerable time introducing us to the clinical trial of a drug called NeuVax by a biopharma company I had never heard of, called Galena. I was familiar with the concept of clinical trials in a general sense, from years of following pharmaceutical and biotech companies in financial markets. I knew that they were risky in terms of side effects and that results were considerably more uncertain than with approved medications. But given our predicament, I was prepared to entertain any and all options. The doctor presented the clinical trial as "another option," but it became clear to me that she was keen to steer us in that direction.

This posed a serious dilemma for me. Nadia left the responsibility of the decision entirely up to me. She was scared and in no condition to conduct research of any kind. She had never wanted to know the medical details of her condition, and she certainly wasn't about to start now. But this was the type of pivotal decision that could make all the difference in Nadia's treatment. Quite literally, a matter of life and death. That weighed on me enormously, and I was petrified of making the wrong decision. I began to research as much as I could about clinical trials in general and about NeuVax in particular. It was not easy. I was online for hours at a time, sometimes in the middle of the night, but there was very little information to be found on either NeuVax or Galena, the maker of the drug. So I reached out to friends everywhere, asking for their opinions.

One of the people I reached out to was Martin Shkreli, who would later become world famous as the "bad boy" of the pharmaceutical industry, referred to in some media circles as "the pharma bro." I had met Martin a few years prior, when he was running a hedge fund called MSMB Capital. At the time I was managing the European equity desk of a British investment bank, and given MSMB's active investments in international pharma companies, we'd developed a relationship with his firm. Martin was young and extremely bright. He seemed to work all hours of the night and even showed us a small corner area in his office where he and his trader would take turns sleeping. They were following hundreds of investment positions all over the world, so no matter what time of day or night, they needed to keep their eyes on things. I had done numerous meetings with Martin and had a very high opinion of him. He seemed to have a limitless knowledge of pharmaceutical products and companies, especially for someone as young as he was. There wasn't a single analyst or industry specialist I put in front of Martin that he didn't blow away. My industry analysts and I seemed to leave every meeting having learned more from him than he had from us. Our relationship was friendly, and we had even gone out for drinks on a couple of occasions. So in my information-gathering efforts, I felt comfortable enough to reach out to Martin for his opinion.

This turned out to be a blessing. Martin ran through the risks of clinical trials in general and pointed out that "sponsors" (doctors who recruit patients for a trial) are compensated for each patient they bring in. This posed obvious (and somewhat shocking) ethical conflicts of interest that I had not been aware of, and that our oncologist had not disclosed, at least as far as we could recall. He also noted that Galena was a company with a $300 million market capitalization but with virtually no operating income and some $30 million in cash on its balance sheet. The rest was *goodwill* (known in finance as an intangible asset). He noted that the shareholder list comprised individuals and was devoid of a single accredited pharmaceutical institution or recognized pharmaceutical investor.

All of this made me uncomfortable. These factors, in combination with other data points I was able to collect, mostly relating to the physical demands of the trial, led us to our final decision to skip the clinical trial. In retrospect, this was the right thing to do. Galena was subsequently the center of a widely reported stock-fraud case involving the manipulation of its share price. And in 2016 the company discontinued the phase III trial of our version of NeuVax (called PRESENT) on the basis of futility, based on a report by the Independent Data Monitoring Committee.

Think what you may of the pharma bro's later trials and tribulations. But I am grateful to this day for the time and advice he afforded us.

Spinning Class Part Two

A couple of weeks after dealing with the clinical-trial decision, our doctor informed us that she was relocating to Hawaii and that she would transfer our care to Sloan Kettering. Given that we were already contemplating a second opinion, we welcomed her suggestion and thanked her for the referral. We were pretty excited about moving the treatment there. Sloan Kettering is renowned for its expertise and research, and it is often described as the best clinic in the world for cancer care.

Our new oncologist (also an Asian American woman) had her own little stage act. There was always a sense of buildup or anticipation before she walked into the room. And when she met with us, she was always surrounded by her staff. They all seemed to tiptoe around her as if to project her

as the "guru" or "grand master" of ceremonies.
They deployed strange communication techniques
designed to make the patient feel better and to
encourage patient communication. For instance,
when my wife was speaking, nobody ever inter-
jected or interrupted. And if one of the team were
speaking to Nadia, they would immediately go
quiet the second my wife opened her mouth. They
also had a strange way of looking straight at her
when she spoke. There was no room for distractions
or nonsense. The focus was always entirely on the
patient. As far as they were concerned, the spouse
wasn't even in the room. It was clear that this was
a deliberate tactic, and surely a product of much
research and consideration. But I never understood
why they would altogether ignore the input of the
caregiver, which is what I believed they were doing.
My comments or interjections evoked nothing
in terms of response. Their eyes would turn back
immediately to the patient as if I had said nothing
at all. Surely I, the spouse, who spent 24/7 with the
patient, would know a little something about how
she was feeling or reacting to a certain medication.

I also knew a little something about how Nadia
was interpreting their comments. And more
importantly, I was in a position to expose Nadia if
she were *misleading* them. In other words, Nadia's

wish to feel better, and to constantly pretend things were better than they were, would sometimes compel her to say misleading things.

"So, how have you been feeling, Nadia? How is your cough?"

"A little better, actually."

Bullshit. I was the one with her all night, every night, listening to her cough and witnessing her discomfort. It bothered me that our new doctor and her team would take the patient at face value for every word, not suspecting or intuiting she may be deluding herself. Surely the caregiver had some valuable information to contribute, no?

I am not a doctor or psychologist, but to this day I question why medical professionals would apply the same "template" to all patients, given how differently each patient may interpret or respond to a consultation. My input, of course, would not have made a difference in the ultimate outcome. After all, Nadia's condition was terminal. But my feedback may have been useful in terms of administering medications to alleviate her symptoms or discomfort. In any case, and for whatever reason, I never felt like my input was welcome.

All that said, our oncologist and her team were extremely professional and, no doubt, experts in their field. They knew every detail of Nadia's medical history and were up to date on every aspect of her treatment.

And yet even in the ultraprofessional setting of the world's best cancer clinic, the spin factor was ever present. For example, when doctors perform CT scans on cancer patients, the results are compared to the prior CT scan to assess disease progression. While at Sloan Kettering, one of Nadia's fairly frequent chest infections prompted the doctors to perform a CT of her torso. The new scan showed two differences relative to the prior scan. First, it showed that the tumors in her chest had reduced in both size and number. This was obviously great news, as it meant that some or all of the tumors were responding to the treatment. The scan, however, also revealed several tumors in her liver "suspicious for hepatic metastases" that were not present in the prior scan. This was obviously very bad news. The median survival of a patient with liver metastases is about *half* that of someone with only lung metastases. The only metastases that predict a shorter median survival than those in the liver are brain metastases. *Surely this would be something the oncologist would highlight, right?*

Wrong.

There was only a fleeting mention of the liver at the end of the meeting. The emphasis was square

on the progress observed in the lungs. And once
again Nadia walked away with a far more positive
message than I believe corresponded to the report.
Eventually, they would have no choice but to come
clean and bring the patient up to speed, but they
would wait as long as possible.

I never agreed with this approach, but I eventually figured out its twisted logic. If a patient has
a limited amount of time left to live, why not give
them as many good days as possible? What would
be the point of giving them bad news if it wasn't
absolutely necessary? *I understood the logic behind
it, but I always felt it would make the final discussion
all the more difficult. How do you go from "things
are progressing well" to "you have a few months or
weeks left to live"?*

It felt to me as if the burden of bad news was
somehow being transferred to me. If they weren't
going to keep the patient up to speed as to her real
condition, then it would presumably be up to me to
do so. After all, this charade had consequences. It
makes a material difference for a terminal patient
to know where they truly stand. Without making
light of this, it goes without saying that leaving this
world and all that you know and love behind is a
pretty big deal—to put it mildly. A patient needs
time to accept and digest what is happening to

them. And depending on the patient's nature and condition, they may require more or less time to come to terms with it, and therefore more or less time to put their emotional and life affairs in order. I understood the "more happy days" logic the Sloan Kettering team seemed to be applying. But it had consequences for Nadia and for me. Her acknowledgment of her real timeline was being postponed, in a way. And the brutal burden of catching her up to reality was left to me—*as if I didn't have enough on my plate.*

The Middle

When your partner has been diagnosed with a terminal illness, your life is plunged into a very strange *middle*. You can no longer live your old life, because everything has changed. Your work schedule is altered to accommodate your medical obligations. Your holidays are pretty much out the window, because your spouse's condition is highly unpredictable and usually incompatible with flights or long journeys. For extended periods of time you are no longer able to do even simple things like go out to dinner or go to a movie. But even activities

you *can* do on your own, like going for a run or listening to music, you rarely feel like doing.

I loved exercising and going for long runs once
or twice a week. But the emotional strain of dealing
with Nadia's condition drained me to a point that I
just didn't *feel* like doing anything. In part because
I couldn't quite *enjoy* anything anymore. I used to
also enjoy going out with my friends, drinking up a
storm, and talking and laughing late into the night.
We would even go on weekend trips to other cities
and party like college kids. But when you are living
your spouse's condition day to day, you are simply
too depressed to do any of those things. It's as if a
large cloud was hanging over my head all the time,
and all my energy was sapped. As a consequence, I
stopped exercising, put on weight, and started feeling depressed more often than not.

At the same time, you know that your life will
soon be very different because your partner won't
be around much longer. And as unpleasant and
confusing as it is to envision that new life, you
can't help but do it from time to time. You think
about what kind of job you can manage once you
will have to devote much more time to your children. You think about whether it's better to stay in
the same house or same town, or whether it would
be better for you and the kids to get a fresh start

somewhere else. You wonder what your emotional life will be like when your wife of twenty years is no longer there. You wonder what types of hobbies or activities you'll want to pursue once your free time is yours and not *ours*. But as much as you may try to envision that future life, you are not actually there yet. So you're basically stuck in a strange *middle*. And you have no idea how long you will be there.

Living in this middle led me to experience frequent bouts of extreme anxiety. I found myself feeling restless all the time, and I constantly felt as if I had lost control of my life entirely. Everything revolved around my wife's condition: if and when I went to work, what we did on weekends, what we ate for dinner, *everything*. This was extremely draining for me during those long, agonizing months. And from time to time the pressure became too much.

The Pressure Cooker

As the mental pressure and physical exhaustion built during these months, I would occasionally slip into periods of self-destruction. Maybe it was the feeling of helplessness that despite my every effort, I was unable to change things? Maybe it was the frustration of being on the receiving end of Nadia's regular outbursts and not being able to fight back? Maybe it was the guilt I was feeling about the times I'd made her unhappy in the past? Or the frustration that I was caught in a long, drawn-out drama I'd never chosen to be in and never wanted for her? Or maybe it was the sense of helplessness that for the first time in my life *I couldn't solve her problem.* Whatever it was, it was chewing away at me, and I dealt with it the only way I knew how—by indulging in my own version of *self-destruction.*

I had always been a big drinker. But not the stereotypical drinker that leaps to mind when I say this. I never was a nasty drunk. I didn't get mean or violent. On the contrary, alcohol made me silly and funny, and sometimes a little crazy (but "good" crazy). For me, alcohol was always just a part of life. Having lived in Europe for long periods at a time, I was raised in the more tolerant and moderate European mind-set around drinking. I would spend my summers in Spain and France, and I got used to going out and drinking from a very young age (fifteen or sixteen). It was all considered normal back then. We would stay out late with friends, especially in summer, and that usually involved drinking. As a result, I developed a pretty high tolerance for alcohol and a healthy "demystified" attitude toward it. In my later years, when I started working in New York, my bosses were old-school Brits in the finance business. Anybody who has any recollection of the finance industry in the '90s, and knows anything about the English, will understand the picture I am trying to paint here. These guys drank every single day, either with clients or just to hang out. As the junior guy in the team, I had to tag along. Yet despite being the youngest, I was usually the one flopping bodies into limos at the end of the day.

So when Nadia's cancer hit, I leaned far too heavily on the booze. I was still getting up early and doing my job. But the combination of long working hours, very little sleep, and the emotional stress I was enduring was too much for me. I slipped into a pattern where the drinking was as much an outlet as it was a source of energy. And it wasn't just drinking. Without dwelling too much on the specifics, I started doing things only college students should do. Sometimes I needed something to help me fall asleep. Sometimes I needed something to help me wake up. And sometimes I just wanted to escape. Alcohol seemed to cover all of these pretty well.

For example, when you are hungover and you have the proverbial "hair of the dog," you feel better almost right away. If you are sober and then have, say, three or four drinks, you feel very lucid at first. Your mind seems to work more quickly than it normally does. And you seem to have more energy. But if you keep drinking, you eventually pass out, and so you manage to sleep. And of course, while you are under the influence of alcohol, you manage to escape, or at least temporarily subdue, your stress level. So no matter what handy helpers I was using to manage my energy level and get through the really difficult days, alcohol was always part of the mix.

Needless to say, the body of a forty-six-year-old man is not designed to withstand what I was doing to myself. But it was all just a means of escaping from the nightmare we were in. Naturally, it didn't work. When the alarm went off in the morning, I still had to go to work, and my wife was still a cancer patient. And so I would eventually manage to rein it in. Until the pressure built up again and the pattern repeated.

The Boys

One of the most heart-wrenching and difficult parts of this whole ordeal was handling the communication with our boys. The tragedy we were living affected each of us in a different way. Nadia had to bear the brunt of it all, of course. And not just the physical hardship of being poisoned, burned, and probed, which is basically what chemo, radiation, and multiple operations *are*. She had to deal with the unimaginable trauma of facing death and losing it all. To this day I am dumbfounded at how any human being could process something like that. *Our psyche is conditioned to accept death in old age, not in the prime of our lives.* For my side, I was able to understand all of this because I was an adult. But for my children the experience was altogether different.

Our older son, Ivan, was twelve when his mother was first diagnosed. Like many kids of his generation, he was far smarter than his age would suggest. Luca was eight at the time, and a different personality type altogether. He was the happy-go-lucky one, always smiling but equally perceptive. I have often commented with friends and other parents how remarkable it is that children from the same parents can be so different. They really do come to this world with a little personality of their own. It is truly amazing. And yet, within each of their unique personalities, you can see traits of yourself and of your partner. Ivan was always the quiet, thinking type. He was very sensitive and perceptive but would rarely express his emotions. In this regard Ivan was his own soul (Nadia and I were always very expressive). But despite the quiet demeanor, Ivan had his father's intensity—and his mother's temper! I often imagine what Ivan will be like as an adult. And let's just say, he's not a guy you want to cross. Luca, by contrast, was more easygoing and was no doubt endowed with the "people-pleasing" gene. If EQ (emotional quotient) is a real thing, then Luca's is sky high.

I thought long and hard about how to talk to the boys about their mom's condition. It didn't help that it was fluid and ever changing. Equally, it didn't help that her physical appearance would go through so many contrasting cycles. Children don't understand subtleties as well as adults do. They tend to view things in a black-and-white manner. "Is Mommy okay or not?" "Is Mommy cured or not?" These questions were hard enough to answer as an adult. They were nearly impossible to answer to a child.

I read various articles about how to deal with children when one of the parents is terminally ill. One of the most common questions friends would ask was "How are the children holding up?" I never knew how to answer that. There are competing theories as to how best to handle these types of situations, mostly regarding the manner and timing of communicating something as traumatic as the terminal condition of a parent. Everybody agrees that honesty is important, that death is natural, and that keeping it from children can be detrimental. Sure, but how on earth do you actually come out and say it? My inclination ultimately was to trust my own instinct as a parent, rather than to abide by a script or set of instructions. After all, I knew my children better than anybody. It should be up to me to know when and how much to tell them.

We were always a very communicative and open family. We would sit at the dinner table every night with no distractions (no TV, music, video games, or the like) and just talk and laugh about pretty much anything. We are also not the type of family that keeps things very quiet. Even when Nadia and I fought, the boys could hear us. And one of them would usually volunteer their opinion the next day. "Papa, I know Mama gets a little crazy sometimes, but once you've made your point, you should drop it and stop going around in circles, that just makes things worse."

Because our fights never involved personal insults or excessive profanity, Nadia and I felt comfortable letting them overhear us. We were just arguing, *loudly*. There was never a danger of either of us walking out on the relationship, so the kids didn't really have anything to fear. In fact, we kind of thought it was healthy for the kids to see us fighting and resolving things. I wanted them to understand that relationships (especially marriages) can be difficult. That no one partner gets to dominate the other. That it's okay to disagree and stand up for yourself. I have seen plenty of domineering wives (and husbands) in my life, and that's not what I want my boys to think marriage is about. But most importantly, I wanted them to understand that no matter what the argument was about or how heated it got, Mama and I still loved each other and would never leave each other.

So against this backdrop of relative transparency, how much would I tell the boys? As it turned out, you can't plan out something like this with any accuracy. The kids are bound to overhear conversations—and even if they don't, *they just have a way of knowing.* Which isn't to say I didn't make a concerted effort. After all, it was my job to keep everybody on the Happy Express.

But when Nadia's cancer returned that summer, just months after she finished her first-line treatments, the trapeze act became more difficult. It's easy to tell your kids that Mommy is going to be fine when she is getting treated the first time around. Because even though her subtype was aggressive, there was no reason to believe she couldn't recover. In other words, saying "Mommy will be fine" wasn't a lie. *With recurrence, it was.* I could no longer make categorical statements, but instead used conditional words like "should" or "could." Kids notice that sort of thing. So without my telling them explicitly, they started to understand. The fact is, I wasn't prepared to work with the alternative. I was not going to promise my children that their mother was going to be fine when I knew for a fact she wasn't. I don't think they would have ever forgotten or forgiven me for a lie of that magnitude. You can break a promise when it's about Christmas gifts or holidays. Not this.

Eventually, our counselor at Sloan Kettering would help us understand that we *needed* to tell the boys, that we had to prepare them for what was to come. And slowly, in our own way, we would.

The Spiral

In December 2014, some eighteen months after Nadia was first diagnosed with cancer, and about six months after her cancer recurred, things started to get really bad. We were accustomed to post-chemo dips and "steroid crashes" after her treatments, and we often ended up in the emergency room as a consequence. But in December, things would become more definitive.

By this stage of her treatment, Nadia had been through a pretty serious list of chemo drugs, none of which had managed to contain the cancer. In her first-line treatment, after the initial diagnosis, she was treated with AC-T (Adriamycin, cyclophosphamide, and Taxol). And after the cancer returned to her lungs, she went on to carboplatin and Taxotere—which had such severe side effects they had to take her off it. They then administered another chemo drug called Gemcitabine. The first round of treatment seemed fairly tolerable. She felt tired and a little nauseated, but it seemed manageable. Yet for some reason, the second round triggered a major downward spiral. She spent nearly ten days in bed with all sorts of aches and pains and an intermittent fever. She would complain of tightness in her chest, heaviness in her head, and all sorts of bone pains in her back and legs. Eventually it got bad enough that we had to take her to the ER.

They treated her for about a day and managed to make her feel better. Some of the symptoms were due to dehydration, which they were able to quell with IV fluids. So we went back home expecting her recovery to continue. *It didn't.* Things got progressively worse, and her symptoms returned. Less than a week later, we were back at the ER, except this time she would spend a full week in the hospital. They put her on a variety of different antibiotics trying to address her persistent fever. They even had doctors from the infectious-disease team examine her.

After a few days of trying to figure out what was causing the pain and fevers, the doctors finally told us what we had quietly feared all along. *Nadia's symptoms were not caused by a mysterious infection or virus, but rather by the cancer itself.* At this point the cancer had also metastasized to the bones and was causing the random pains in her back and legs. And the fever was due to the spread of the cancer itself; it was the body's reaction to the tumor growth, referred to as "tumor fever." The bone metastasis itself was not any more alarming than the lung recurrence. In fact, metastasis to the bones has a longer survival duration than metastasis to the lungs. But the cancer to the bones would throw an array of new pains and medications into the mix.

I left the hospital that Thursday night fearing we had very little time left. She had lost a huge amount of weight and was in constant pain and discomfort. For the first time since this ordeal began, she actually looked like somebody whose time was running out. She was barely able to make it to the bathroom on her own, only to collapse back into the hospital bed. She wouldn't eat or drink at all and seemed to get weaker by the day. I knew the cancer was spreading quickly and that her latest scan, only three weeks before, had been horrific, citing cancer in the lungs, bones, and liver. I feared the worst and needed answers. I was tired of playing the "positive spin" game. Everything I was seeing with my own two eyes suggested that things were really bad. I was no longer willing to bite my tongue.

The following morning, before going back to the hospital to see Nadia, I called the oncologist's office and asked to speak to our doctor directly. I told her I was very concerned about Nadia's condition, that I had read the latest scan and that, though I was not a doctor, I knew things were pretty bad. I demanded to know what the state of play was and if it was necessary for me to call relatives at this point. We knew the cancer had spread. Her condition was worse than ever, and I believed she looked like she had very little time left.

"Doctor, she does not look to me like somebody who has more than a few days left. You need to be honest with me. What's going on?" I implored.

"Yes, it is a cancer that's moving fast," she admitted. "Do you want to have a time range? Is that what you're asking?"

"Yes—are we looking at days here?" I replied.

"No, not days. In the best case, we can manage to try some third-line treatments and buy us a couple of months here or there," she offered. "If we keep her on steroids and nothing else works, the worst-case scenario could be as little as a month."

Given what I had learned about doctors and their communication strategies, and knowing the state my wife was in, it seemed to me that we were looking at the shorter end of that range. I was also very concerned that Nadia wasn't entirely conscious of how little time she had left. I had reached my limit. I could no longer tolerate the spinning.

"Doctor, I know that we're meeting with you later today. You should be aware that Nadia does not understand what her timeline really is. This morning she told me she thought she had three years left. I don't know where she got that number, given where we are, but that's what she seems to believe. She is clinging on to that. Just be aware."

"I understand," the doctor replied. "I will speak to her."

I hung up and collapsed onto the sofa. My legs were shaking and I felt like vomiting. I knew the end was near. And I was petrified of what lay ahead.

Telling Her

So there we were. My wife still believed she had a few years left. Despite feeling the way she did and in the face of the overwhelming evidence of deterioration in her most recent scan. I knew I had to leave it up to the oncologist to come clean with her prognosis. And I knew how difficult it would be for Nadia to accept.

Later that afternoon, the doctor visited us as promised. She greeted us both with a hug and sat down next to Nadia's bed. I took the chair on the other side of the room to give them the privacy they needed. After about thirty minutes of mostly medical talk, Nadia finally (and uncharacteristically) confronted the elephant in the room.

"So, Doctor, what does all this mean for me?"

The doctor extended her hand and held Nadia's. She was speaking in a soft and caring voice. "Nadia, we have not been able to stop the progression of the disease. We've tried a number of agents, but it has spread. The way you've been feeling these last few days was due to the cancer, not an infection of any sort. In the best case, we can try to treat you, and hopefully we can get a few more months—"

Before she could finish her sentence, Nadia burst into tears. *I will never forget the look of fear and panic in her eyes.* She looked right at me, as if begging for an alternative interpretation of what she had just heard. I had always been her last bastion of support, her caretaker, the problem solver, the one person in her life who could always make things better. But this time I knew I couldn't. There was no magic trick up my sleeve, no alternative answer for me to offer. I moved close to her and held her hand. But I couldn't stand to see her cry, to see the helplessness in her eyes. I had to look down and try to contain my own tears, which of course I could not.

She finally gathered herself enough to ask, "But Doctor, I thought I had two or three years left."

"No, Nadia, not years. Not years," she said in a gentle tone.

Nadia couldn't stop crying, and the doctor could see this was no time to discuss the worst-case scenario that she had mentioned to me prior to the meeting. That would have to wait for another time. We both understood that what Nadia had just been told was more than enough for her to digest, at least for now.

Magic Pills

I stayed with Nadia until late that evening. The following morning I called Nadia to tell her I was on my way over. But much to my surprise, she sounded much better—not just emotionally but physically. She went on to tell me that she would be released that day and could go home with me. *What?* I was absolutely shocked. She had barely been able to speak the prior day. She had been in terrible shape all week. She'd been frail and had trouble just getting out of bed. *How on earth could they send her home? And how could she be sounding so much better?*

When I got to the hospital, she wasn't lying in bed but rather sitting in a chair in the corner eating her breakfast, smiling, and speaking to one of the nurses. *I couldn't believe what I was seeing.* The previous evening, she couldn't even move. One of our dear friends, who had also been with her the prior day, was utterly stunned when we told her Nadia was going to be released. *It was truly incredible.*

What I had not yet learned was the extent to which doctors are able to revive patients, even critically ill ones, at least for a limited period of time. In Nadia's case, they had administered a steroid called dexamethasone. I would later come to learn, through research of my own, that a great part of the malaise she had been feeling in the past week or so was caused by tumor-induced inflammation. Steroids act as an anti-inflammatory that also gives patients strength and fuels their appetite. And these things are, of course, circular. The more someone can eat, the more strength they have, which in turn makes them more active and then more hungry. Moreover, the steroids also helped mask the bone pain and fever.

Nadia's turnaround was remarkable. Of course, the underlying disease was still on the move—nothing to date had managed to slow its progress. But from a clinical standpoint (i.e., how she looked and felt), she was a different person. She was talking, eating, and walking around in a way we hadn't seen in weeks.

The fact that Nadia could come home was a blessing for which we will be eternally grateful. It allowed us to enjoy Christmas as a family and spend New Year's Eve with some of our dear friends. I was even able to take her into the city to spend a night in a nice hotel. We had to monitor her energy levels carefully, but we were able to go to dinner and even take a short walk afterward.

But as miraculous as the steroids were, I knew they couldn't last forever. She would remain on the steroids chronically from that point on. The doctors knew her body couldn't survive another "steroid crash," the dramatic drop in energy she experienced if she suddenly stopped taking them. But how long they could keep her on them, without significant side effects or her body getting used to them, I did not know. We would simply try to enjoy every minute of every day for as long as they seemed to work.

All of that said, I still believe to this day that the doctors should have done a better job of warning us of this "rebound" effect. As fortunate as we were to have had that final period with Nadia in relatively good health, it was a very confusing time for me and for those around her, because none of us expected it. It was made increasingly confusing because the steroid treatment was accompanied by low doses of a third-line chemo agent called eribulin. Third-line chemo treatments are used for patients who have tried at least two previous chemotherapy combinations unsuccessfully. Eribulin was a relatively new drug. In the phase III clinical trial called EMBRACE, the use of eribulin had managed to extend median survival by two and a half months (from 10.6 months to 13.1). It was just effective enough to be approved and used—but it was obviously not a game changer in any significant way. And yet the doctors always gave Nadia the impression that the treatment itself was the primary reason behind the remarkable rebound, not the steroids. *I knew that was bullshit.* They had not administered any eribulin until at least a week after her miraculous exit from the hospital. The bounce was entirely a response to the steroids, literally from one day to the next. But this all fed into the hope the doctors were always supposed to provide.

The Office

This all made things very difficult to explain to family, friends, and colleagues. It was great that she was feeling better. And all we wanted was for her to have as much quality time as possible. *But people's conception of a terminally ill cancer patient is linear: they are supposed to go from bad to worse, not rebound magically from one day to the next.* I myself didn't understand it at first. But the fact was, she was up and about and feeling better. And even though I knew it was not sustainable indefinitely, we would try to enjoy her newfound strength as much as possible.

During the week that Nadia had spent in the hospital, I had tried to go back to work. I was feeling self-conscious about how much time I was spending out of the office, especially because my firm was still paying me. The day I went in, my boss asked me how Nadia was doing. I replied candidly that she was doing terribly. She was in the hospital and in pretty bad shape.

Later that morning, after my bosses had time to speak to each other about my situation, they came back to me and told me, in no uncertain terms, that I should go back to the hospital and take care of my wife. In addition to their sense of decency and compassion, they also knew it would be impossible for me to concentrate on work as long as Nadia was in this condition. We had put a coverage plan in place so that two of my colleagues would be in charge of my clients in my absence. By all accounts they had been doing a good job. We also all understood that this was not the type of job you could float in and out of. In addition to the daily research and marketing trips we were hosting throughout North America, we had many live transactions going on all day long. You had to be on top of everything in case your clients asked about any one of the many balls we had in the air. Unless you were immersed in it on a continuous day-to-day basis, you were pretty much out of the loop. I understood that my trying to periodically take the reins, only to disappear again at the next medical crisis, was disruptive to the group and to the flow of business.

So I continued to spend time at home, helping out with the boys and taking care of Nadia. I would occasionally check in with my bosses, who continued to insist I take care of my family ("It's what matters most") and that I shouldn't worry about work ("Let us take care of that"). They also knew that the issue of medical insurance was absolutely critical. At this stage, my back-of-the-envelope calculations estimated that since Nadia's initial diagnosis, her various treatments, operations, and emergency-room and hospital visits had generated expenses somewhere in the region of $1.5 to $2 million. Our insurance had covered pretty much everything. My bosses were not about to throw us to the lions in the circumstance we were in.

In any case, we considered ourselves blessed to have the firm's unconditional support. To this day, I don't quite know how to repay them. They allowed me to spend my wife's last weeks and months with her, be it at home or in the hospital. It afforded me invaluable time with my children, who needed to feel the additional support and security of their healthier parent more than ever.

I eventually sent out an email to the entire firm, copying all of my clients, thanking my bosses for their extraordinary generosity. They deserved all the recognition in the world, not just internally but from the very clients that buttered our bread.

Head Doctors and Elephants

Having had the difficult discussion with our oncologist about Nadia's timeline, just prior to the dexamethasone "rally," Sloan Kettering was quick to volunteer a counselor and psychiatrist to make sure we had some emotional support. Our counselor, Dianne, was warm and funny, with extensive experience helping couples in our circumstances. Nadia and I had often tried to discuss delicate matters, but we would always fall into the same pattern. I would eventually say something she didn't want to hear, and she would get upset.

Having Dianne in those conversations was critical. She forced each of us to listen and understand the other's concerns. She would speak to us individually as well, to make sure we could be totally open about our thoughts and feelings. And she would use our group conversations to help bridge any major gaps she perceived between us. These sessions were also critical in that they forced Nadia to discuss and accept where she was. Her natural inclination all along had been to hide from reality. Every step of the way was made more difficult because she simply didn't want to know or accept what was going on. But lying to herself and even to me was easy. She knew I would never say anything too harsh. This had been the case all along. Every headache or cough had to be something other than cancer: "I have a weird tickle in my throat. I must have slept with my mouth open." She would make these comments knowing that I wouldn't state the obvious. The elephant was always in the room, but she knew I wouldn't point at it. I knew the impact my words might have, so I kept them to myself. *And my silence would only serve to vindicate her delusion.*

The truth is, her cancer had spread everywhere. Any ailment or pain was probably related to it. But she never wanted to believe that. And I couldn't find it in me to remind her. So every time I *didn't* say, "No, my love, you have tumors everywhere, that's why your throat tickles," she could carry on believing her own lies.

But this wasn't possible with third parties. When Dianne spoke to us, Nadia would have to come clean, *or at least pretend to.* It was an incredibly twisted game. She could lie to herself, muscle me into shutting up, but pretend to be in touch with reality to anybody who might call her bluff. So we would fade in and out of acceptance, always at her rhythm.

The Headless Chicken

So from mid-December on, when Nadia was released from the hospital, I was basically at home full time. As bad as I felt about not going to work, I knew that there was no circumstance in which I *shouldn't* be with her. If she was feeling well, I should be there to enjoy those moments. After all, neither of us knew how many more good days we would have together. And if she wasn't feeling well, I would need to be there to take care of her and help out with day-to-day chores.

My days would begin at six a.m., when I would make breakfast for the boys, help my little one with his last bits of homework, and then take each of them to school at different starting times. They were close enough to walk themselves, but in the dead of a New York winter, I wasn't going to let them. I would then come home, take care of any administrative issues that were required, go shopping, and ask Nadia what else she needed me to do that day. At 2:45 p.m. I would go back to school to pick up the boys and later help Luca with his homework and heat up dinner. After dinner, I would clean up the dining room and kitchen and watch TV with the family before getting everybody to bed.

But the daily routines never turned out to be as easy as that. They were always interspersed with a million other small chores: return these plates to that neighbor, drop off one of the kids at some party, or practice, or game, or rehearsal. And Nadia's heavy breathing didn't allow her to go up and down the stairs with much ease. So anytime she forgot anything anywhere, I was running up and down a four-story townhouse for her. It was overwhelming at times. I tried not to show my frustration with the endless requests, given Nadia's condition, but it wasn't easy. There was always something. "I left my phone in the basement." "Bring me some water." "My pills are in the bedroom." "Shut off the kids' lights."

It was nonstop.

I knew I was doing the right thing, of course. I was taking care of my wife. I wouldn't have had it any other way. And I did it with all the love in my heart. But it was nothing short of exhausting. And the requests always seemed to coincide with my sitting or lying down. The second I fell into a chair or bed, it would come. Sometimes I could swear it was by design—as if I was constantly being tested to prove my love, or so it seemed. And any rolling of the eyes or subtle sigh on my part would set her off.

Most of the time, I was really only reacting to the lack of forethought going into our movements in and around the house. I felt like most of the requests were perfectly avoidable. If you're going downstairs, take your phone. If you go down for lunch and you know you have to take some of your pills with lunch, bring them down with you. Instead, I would make two separate trips upstairs, when we could have managed with neither. None of these things were a big deal individually, but they sure piled up. Eventually it would be up to me to think ahead. Like a test monkey getting shocked, I eventually caught on. Again, it wasn't that I resented looking after my ailing wife, never. It was the *unnecessary* tasks that got under my skin.

Of course, Nadia didn't mean to do any of this. She was deeply frustrated she couldn't go upstairs and get the stuff herself, the twelve or fifteen times a day she would forget something. And I know she found it even more frustrating to have to ask me to do it, to have to *depend* on me for almost everything. Either way, this was a constant during the months after December 2014.

This may sound petty in the broader context. After all, what Nadia was facing was beyond description. How could I possibly complain? But this is one of the truly difficult issues I believe caregivers face. You care deeply for the person you are helping. But at the end of the day, you are not superhuman, although you're expected to be so every day. You can't show your fatigue or express your frustration, and you can never fail in your duties. And even privately, the mere thought of feeling frustrated or tired engenders a feeling of guilt. It was a very lonely place to be, and it bred in me a renewed respect for persons who dedicate their lives to helping others.

Sex and Stephen Hawking

I remember watching *The Theory of Everything* sometime around February 2015. It was about the life of Stephen Hawking, the world-famous physicist who changed the way we think about the universe. In the movie, Stephen falls in love with a beautiful young lady while he's still healthy. The movie portrays his soon-to-be wife as madly in love with him as well. When he eventually develops his debilitating illness (Lou Gehrig's disease), she demonstrates a steadfast and unconditional will to help him, no matter what. Nothing can keep them apart, and they intend to fight the disease together. It's love as it should be.

But as the movie progresses, Stephen's care becomes ever more demanding. His survival repeatedly surpasses his doctor's expectations, even as his physical condition continues to deteriorate. The pressures on his wife continue to build. And with the passage of time, she eventually seeks solace in another young man, portrayed as a family friend and member of their church.

As I watched the movie, I remember thinking to myself how most viewers would see this. Here he is, dying a slow death, and off she goes with someone else in private. Even my boys, who were watching the movie with me, commented, "But Papa, he's so sick. Is she really going with that other guy? That's not very nice." And under any other circumstance, I would have had exactly the same reaction.

And while I could sympathize with Mrs. Hawking's predicament, I can say with my hand on my heart that I never went that route. I was never exactly a saint, don't get me wrong. But I knew that if there was ever a time to show restraint and respect, this was it. My marital life hadn't been terribly sexual prior to Nadia's illness. After all, twenty years is a long time. But if the sex was minimal before my wife's diagnosis, it was obviously going to be nonexistent afterward.

Still, I knew that if cheating was disrespectful and hurtful under normal circumstances, it was downright insulting under these. Instead I used my friends for emotional support. And given my circumstances, I didn't have much of a libido to worry about anyway. After all, I rarely felt like doing anything at all most of the time, least of all *fucking*.

But all that said, I could see where Mrs. Hawking was coming from. I understood, or at least had *some* understanding of, how she may have felt. I could identify with the physical and emotional erosion of committing unconditionally and *interminably* to a very sick loved one. I turned to my sons and replied, *"I know, boys. That's not a very nice thing to do. But things must be pretty tough for her too."*

'Roid Rage

A few weeks into the dexamethasone treatment, some of the nastier side effects of the steroids started to come into play. Nadia had always been a pretty temperamental person, but after a few weeks on the dexamethasone, she was experiencing full-blown "'roid rage." She became incredibly irritable and would have crazy outbursts. She was displaying an underlying anger that seemed to grow in intensity with each passing week. During these episodes she could be downright mean. And whatever the issue was, her anger was always directed at me (and sometimes at the kids). She would be charming and funny with her friends, but the second the door closed, she'd do a complete 180. She was genuinely hurtful on a number of occasions, and it made helping her all the harder. Here I was doing everything in my power to make her feel better, and all I got in return were earsplitting outbursts and a variety of objects hurled at me for no reason whatsoever. This was extremely difficult for me to digest.

They say there are different types of patients, and Nadia had morphed into the really horrible kind. All of this made me start to feel angry myself. How could anybody be so hurtful and ungrateful at a time like this? Wouldn't this be a good time to try to come to peace with what was happening? To find appreciation for the life you've had and all the people who have loved you?

Once again, I think the doctors did an inadequate job of communicating the risks of the medication they were administering. Had she been warned she might get 'roid rage, she may have been more able to control some of her actions and words. I know I would have certainly benefited from a warning or a heads-up. But nobody offered us that information, so we were caught off guard. As the weeks passed, her rage-fueled episodes became ever more frequent and intense. The children began to suffer from it as well. There was a constant tension in the air. We all walked on eggshells because we knew even the smallest thing would set her off. She projected a combination of intense frustration, anger, and jealousy. Nadia had always been a somewhat controlling person, and her inability to control her surroundings, in combination with the meds, was making her crazy.

On the couple of occasions where I tried to put my foot down, she would yell at me in a way no husband deserved, much less one who was working tirelessly for his wife. I would tell her to stop and that I didn't deserve to be spoken to in such a manner. But it only made things worse. So, for days and weeks, I would live in quiet fear, hoping each day would pass without a major blowup. This was an extremely difficult and lonely time for me. *I was doing the best I could. But privately, in those moments, I just wanted it all to end.*

Stock Markets and White Picket Fences

It is in crisis situations or a circumstance of duress when one's true nature is revealed. My father used to always say that sooner or later, a person will paint his own portrait. In these moments, you'll need to make difficult decisions that will define your character, show who you really are. And, as he would regularly remind me, sometimes the picture turns out well, and sometimes people paint a very ugly portrait of themselves. We had a variety of experiences with a long list of friends during Nadia's illness. And I'm glad to say that, for the most part, the portraits we watched our friends paint were beautiful.

We had made our return to New York in 2008, having left the city six years prior. Our first stint in the Big Apple had lasted around seven or eight years, and during that time, we had always lived right in the city—first in a rental apartment in Murray Hill, and later on the Upper West Side, after buying our first apartment on Columbus Avenue. Our lifestyle in those days was fairly uncomplicated. We didn't have children, and I was earning more than my age or skills warranted. So we did what any young couple in those circumstances would do. We went out with friends constantly. We took great vacations around the world and bought all the flashy stuff only a young couple could think they needed. It was the stereotypical investment-banking lifestyle of the 1990s in the finance capital of the world.

In the intervening years, when we moved to Madrid and Miami, we also enjoyed the city life. In Madrid we rented a spectacular old-school apartment in the city center. It had two living rooms, very high ceilings with old chandeliers, four bedrooms, and servant quarters where our live-in maid stayed. We were right smack in the middle of one of Madrid's prime residential areas, Barrio

Salamanca, surrounded by great restaurants and shops, with everything in walking distance.

Later, in Florida, we would once again live the good city life. I had purchased a condo a few years before in one the nicest buildings in Miami, the Murano at Portofino, nestled in a quiet corner of Miami Beach's South of Fifth area. We were on the twelfth floor with 180-degree views from our balcony, spanning from the city's harbor all the way east to the ocean.

You could look straight ahead and see Fisher Island, separated from us by a canal where cruise ships sailed by each afternoon. The building was top-of-the line everything, with a private elevator entering into the foyer of our apartment (there were no hallways in our tower). And the location was, once again, spectacular. We had shops and restaurants nearby, the beach was a hundred yards away, and we could walk the boys to school. We had plenty of friends in Miami as well, whom we would get together with on a regular basis. Some we had known previously, and others we made very quickly during our time there, either through my work or the boys' school.

But when my work circumstances in Miami changed, I knew we would probably have to return to New York. After all, that was where my old industry was located, and it was where all my old colleagues and clients *still* were. And it was where pretty much every firm in the world was set up. So little by little, we prepared our return. But compared to our first New York stint, our circumstances were now very different. In fact, the world was very different.

For starters, we now had two young boys, ages three and seven. And Nadia and I had never believed children of that age would benefit much from living in New York City. Which isn't to say many parents don't make it work; there are plenty. But I remember being a little boy. I'm pretty sure I would not have wanted to live right smack in the middle of one of the largest, loudest, most congested cities in the world. For all of the Big Apple's wonders and charms, my boys were a little too young to go to Lincoln Center to catch a symphony. So this time we decided to look for a home in the surrounding suburbs. Our days of living the good city life had come to an end.

In addition to the issue of the boys, there was also the small matter of the near meltdown of the global financial markets. The world was coming out of one of the worst crises ever, one that had threatened to throw us all back to the Stone Ages. As I have often explained to friends who are not in the financial industry, the world came close to the brink. We came very near to a situation where if you tried to get money out of an ATM at your bank (where you believed you had savings), the bank could have shown you a zero balance. Have that happen to enough people and you can imagine the ensuing anarchy. It was a scary time for everybody, and it would forever change not just the nature of global finance and the regulatory regime around it, but also its corporate culture and the risk tolerances of companies and investors alike.

So with a renewed sense of caution, Nadia flew to New York for a week to find a good suburban town for us to relocate to. My office-to-be was very near Grand Central, so I told her to start by checking out Connecticut and Westchester County, both of which have beautiful towns with great schools and easy commutes into the city. And this time we wouldn't be looking for a flashy condo or sprawling mansion, but rather something financially savvy and convenient for everybody. We settled on a little town in Westchester County called Bronxville. It was smaller than many of the surrounding towns, but it was known for its great schools and easy commute into the city. Our children would attend an excellent public school, and our purchase of a townhome (versus a huge family home) would ensure we didn't have to pay massive property taxes or incur enormous maintenance expenses. It was a clean, safe little town, the quintessential white-picket-fence town where we would begin our new life.

Self-Portraits

But back to the self-portraits. We had very few friends when we first moved to Bronxville. There was one couple we had met many years ago through a mutual friend, back in the day. But other than the McBrides, who by now had three kids of their own, we were pretty much alone. With the passage of time, it was frankly amazing how many wonderful friends we would make in this new place. I was always at work and constantly reconnecting with dozens of my old friends and clients in the city. But it is a testament to Nadia's magnetic personality how she blossomed in this small, tightly knit town.

Over the course of a few years we made many lifelong friends. And never were the strengths of Nadia's friendships more visible than during the course of her illness. The displays of warmth and generosity were nothing short of extraordinary. When Nadia was too weak to leave the bed (much less cook) after her chemo sessions, her friends would set up a dinner-delivery schedule as well as drop off the kids' lunches during the week. So every other day, one of them would come by with dinner for the family and lunch packs for the boys for their next day at school.

They must have known that I was busy with plenty of other things, or maybe just that I was a terrible cook, but they really stepped up to the plate—no pun intended. Nadia, of course, loved the show of affection and enjoyed seeing her friends every day. Admittedly, I felt a little embarrassed about the whole thing. I could have easily organized for delivery or picked up food from any one of a number of restaurants in the area. But I soon realized that this was a female ceremony of sorts, and I wasn't really supposed to get involved. So I left them to it, content to watch the lovefest go on for weeks and weeks.

It made all the difference in the world to have so much love and support. It was a very difficult time for us, and everybody around us came to our aid. We never felt alone, despite the fact that our families were so far away. We knew we could lean on our friends for any type of help and support, or even just company. I don't know how many of these dear friends—if any—will ever read these pages, but if they ever do, they should know what a difference they made to Nadia's life (and to mine and the boys') in her final weeks and months.

Nadia and I always believed that one's only real legacy in life is how one affects one's surroundings. That every little gesture of kindness matters. That every small act of generosity, every smile, every compliment, every joke, every hug, has an impact. Ultimately the sum of all these small things is what we leave behind. And as minuscule as we are in this vast universe, in a very small way, we make the universe, and our little world, a better place. Our many wonderful friends should know that their acts of kindness made the world a better place. We will be forever grateful for the beautiful portraits they painted of themselves.

The Woman

As I've come to discover over the years, people are rarely black and white, but rather many shades of gray, their lives molded by a variety of experiences, both good and bad. Nadia's upbringing was far more complicated than mine. And many of her personality traits I can trace back to major circumstances or events in her life.

When Nadia was young, she and her family were forced to move from East Pakistan (the country that is now Bangladesh) to Pakistan—after the former became an independent state. Her grandmother on her mother's side was a well-known politician and the first female representative in the Pakistani national assembly. I remember being blown away, on a trip to Toronto to visit her cousins and uncles, when I was shown pictures of Nadia's grandmother (known as Dolly Azad) posing with the likes of Marshal Tito of Yugoslavia, King Hussein of Jordan, Henry Kissinger, and even Mao Zedong.

On the personal side, however, the story is a little less glamorous. Nadia's father abandoned her and her mother when she was a little girl, at around the age of three. Raised by her mother and her uncles in Pakistan and the United Arab Emirates, her fondest childhood memories were of her grandfather's house in Karachi, Pakistan's largest city. She always spoke nostalgically about her time at that house, where she would be spoiled by her grandparents and family servants.

But at the age of seven, Nadia was sent to a boarding school in the mountains of Pakistan. She would spend five years there, in a convent run by Irish nuns, isolated from everyone and everything.

These were very difficult years for her—and, I
believe, formative ones. The decision to send her
there was her mother's, who claims it was the only
thing she could do as a working single parent. I
never bought into this. There are plenty of working
single parents who manage to raise their kids without shipping them off to a mountain. This would
always be a bone of contention between my moth-
er-in-law and myself, and a silent wedge between
Nadia and her mother. Nadia almost never brought
up the subject, and her relationship with her
mother normalized over time. But I knew, from the
rare occasions when we did discuss it, that it was a
scar in their relationship.

It is clear to me that her five years in that convent were transformative, and not in a good way.
On the few occasions she ventured to talk about
that period of her life, it was never in a positive light.
She said it was cold. It was so cold that she developed chilblains in her hands, a condition whereby
continued exposure to cold air creates an inflammation of the blood vessels. This is why her fingers
were always a little swollen (and why it wasn't easy
to buy her rings!).

Otherwise, there was the odd comment now
and then about a horrible sister, referring to one
of the nuns. She also mentioned a bully among the

ranks of interns, who she claimed made her life impossible. Nadia also once told me about being quarantined because she developed the measles. Apparently she spent ten days alone in a room. She joked that the only good thing about those ten days was that she got a pile of comic books to read and didn't have to share a bathroom. She told me very little about her time there, and the only physical description she gave was of a cold, secluded place with long corridors and numerous statues throughout, some of which petrified her at night, depending on how the moonlight hit them.

It all sounded extremely bleak and depressing. And for a little girl away from her family, it must have been terrifying. It speaks volumes how little I actually know about the place, considering she was there for five years, and I was married to her for twenty! It was obvious to me she wanted to erase the experience from her memory. *But nothing is more telling of the place and her circumstances there than how she got out.*

Much like in a prison, any mail was monitored by the nuns. No letter would get in or out of the convent without being checked. After five long years, Nadia pleaded with a security guard to post a letter to her grandfather in Karachi. In the letter she begged him to get her out of there. Luckily for her, the guard agreed and the letter was sent. By all accounts, Nadia's grandfather adored her. She was the apple of his eye. And every conversation I had over the years with her relatives seemed to corroborate that. So you can imagine his reaction to Nadia's letter.

As the story goes, he showed up in person with his driver and made it clear Nadia was to be released immediately. Her family was not as wealthy or powerful as they had been back in the Bangladesh years. I assume they lost everything when they had to move to Pakistan, as many political families do in such circumstances. But I imagine they still commanded a bit of influence. In any case, the nuns had no choice but to let Nadia go home for good that day.

Still, I am convinced all those years alone in a remote boarding school had a profound effect on her. And knowing that her father abandoned her, even more so. Nadia could sometimes behave very defensively. It wouldn't take much to elicit an aggressive response if she thought somebody was attacking or insulting her in any way. She had a strong self-protective instinct, perhaps because she felt she'd always had to fend for herself. She was also very proud and wasn't afraid to ruffle feathers if she thought somebody was demeaning or insulting her. Having been abandoned by her father and semi-abandoned by her mother during her convent years, Nadia had only her grandparents and extended family (cousins, aunts, and uncles). I believe this made her feel like the black sheep of the family and somewhat humiliated at times. I think this is why she fought so hard to defend her pride and self-esteem later in life.

I give Nadia enormous credit for managing to overcome all of those ghosts from her past. Despite everything that she had endured as a largely abandoned child, she was an extraordinary mother. Of all the fights we ever had, none of them ever had anything to do with the kids. Sure, there would be a disagreement here or there about how to discipline them. But I never doubted her as a mother. I knew she appreciated the privilege of being a parent more than I did.

We are all conditioned by our pasts, especially as parents. And in compensating for our pasts, she was a much better parent than me. When she reprimanded the boys, she was usually right. And even if she wasn't, she was so vested emotionally that she *deserved* to be right. I never fought her on these issues, even if I believed she was wrong, because she was never wrong *enough*. Her caring and concern compensated for any small imperfections in her argument. So I supported her, and I was always proud of the kids she was raising. And the kids responded. She taught them respect, manners, and an appreciation for things, all things. If they didn't finish their food, they would hear it. "Do you know how many children in this world would kill to have that food?" It was always dramatic but always true. And I was happy for them to hear it.

Given my rather demanding job, I was away most of the time. So ultimately I always felt *she* was raising them. It couldn't have been easy on her. After all, her past did not warrant a happy-go-lucky attitude toward life. But despite that fact, she managed to raise the boys with plenty of laughter and joy.

Like many parents who aren't there 24/7, my longing to see the boys blinded me to any possible imperfections in their behavior. It was always heaven for me just to be with them. Before Ivan was born, I had no idea how powerful a parent's love for their child could be. It is simply unlike any other type of love you will ever feel. If your range of emotions was once between one and ten, with children it becomes negative ten to positive twenty. You feel stress and concern the likes of which you never imagined before, but also a happiness you couldn't dream of prior to having them. You can fall in love with a woman, but your relationship with her will always be "adult" and therefore always a little complicated. No matter how much you love that person, there will always be issues and she will always be imperfect. The same can be said of a relationship with a sibling or a parent. But the love you feel for a child is pure and totally unconditional. And it never wears off. *The joy I feel when I see my boys in the morning is the same every day. It never declines, no matter how many years go by and how old they grow.*

Of course, for Nadia the boys were her day-to-day. She loved them just as much as I did and felt the same joy seeing them every morning, but she had to deal with the more real or practical side of things. And there is nothing easy about that. Taking care of the boys is exhausting. I actually made a funny video about it in Miami when Nadia left us for one week to go house hunting in New York. It depicts the boys driving their father nuts in Mommy's absence. It's a ten-minute video collage of the boys fighting, playing video games, complaining about being hungry or thirsty, nagging me to go shopping at Toys "R" Us, and then fighting again. Well, you get the idea.

They say that patterns repeat. That a child who was abused will one day grow up to be an abusive parent. I have never been entirely convinced of that theory. And over the years, Nadia dispelled it entirely. Her father had left her when she was only three. Her mother shipped her off to a remote convent when Nadia was seven because she didn't want *"to wear"* her. Later, she was forced to grow up with her uncles and cousins, some of whom were warm and welcoming and others decidedly not. So in a sense she was always an outsider, even in her own family. Yet Nadia's love and dedication to her children were truly remarkable, given her own childhood. She instinctively knew how to be the kind of parent she never was lucky enough to have.

She eventually repaired her relationship with her mother, by which I mean she eventually forgave her. But nothing was ever really normal for her.

And yet, despite all this, Nadia managed to defy her past. Sure, her reactions were at times hyperbolic or defensive. But she was the best wife and mother any husband could have ever asked for. She adored her boys more than anything in the world. And the young men they are today, and will become, will always be the product of her love and caring.

The Cancer Flu

By mid-February we decided it wasn't worthwhile for me to sit with Nadia at every chemo session. I should clarify. This wasn't "hard-core" chemo, but rather that third-line drug I described earlier. We decided this not because I was getting tired or lazy, or because I didn't care anymore. It was simply because I knew that she was getting something that had virtually no side effects, and whose overall efficacy on metastatic cancer was pretty much (from what I could gather) that of an aspirin. *But more importantly, she preferred me not to be around.*

She had a great relationship with the nurses. The infusions were completely nonintrusive (she already had a meta-port in her chest), so the actual take-in time was minimal. Unlike other chemo agents, this one was injected very quickly. They would chat, and after about thirty minutes she was out of there. This was by far the most forgiving chemo agent she ever received. I also didn't want to join her in these sessions because I grew uncomfortable with the ongoing "cancer bluff."

Nadia was, of course, still on her big steroid high, which lasted much longer than I ever thought possible. So she was feeling much better than back in December, when pretty much everyone thought we

were down to her last few days. But as the steroids
would begin to wear off, she would start to develop
some symptoms of what I believe must have been
the underlying disease. But God forbid anybody
would actually suggest that. When she would complain to the oncologist of knee pain, it couldn't be
the osseous (bone) metastases. No. If her belly was
swollen as if she were pregnant, it couldn't be the
cancer in her liver. No. If she complained of diz-
ziness from time to time, it had to be the meds,
not any of the tumors in the brain. Of course not.
There was always some mysterious alternative
explanation. I also noticed that despite all of these
symptoms, the doctors no longer requested scans.
The last one had been months ago.

So when I'd pick up Nadia from her sessions,
I would ask her how things had gone. And I was
baffled every single time by her response. As far
as I could gather, the oncologist—who had main-
tained a serious end-of-life conversation with my
wife just three months prior (and who knew how
denial-prone my wife was)—would never mention
the C-word again, at least not until the very end. It
was as if Nadia had developed a strange, long-last-
ing flu that had merely *started* as cancer.

Warning Signs

About three years prior, I had traveled to Spain with my brother to visit our uncle, who was dying of cancer. We were told via my mother that he probably didn't have long to live. My brother, who was living in Houston, called me and explained that the situation didn't sound good. We both interrupted our work schedules and traveled mid-week to Madrid. We then took a three-hour train to León, in the northwest of Spain, where my uncle lived. I remembered his condition during our visit, which turned out to be around three months prior to his death. He had a pale complexion and was a little bloated and very weak. He would sleep most of the day and had to make a huge effort just to speak. In March 2015 I began to detect some of these symptoms in Nadia. I knew that with the passage of time, the steroids would stop having an effect. I noticed her breathing getting heavier. And each time she went downstairs to sit in the dining room or living room, her escapades were shorter lived. She would eventually go back to bed to sleep, ever more frequently, and always for longer.

The steroids had done wonders to keep her going and subdue the symptoms of the underlying disease. But as with all drugs, your body eventually gets used to a certain dose and the marginal effect declines with time. You either ramp up the dosage or begin to come off it. During her illness Nadia would always ask me to massage her back. The cancer had spread to her lymphatic system and her thoracic cavity (the area between her abdomen and chest). For some reason this translated into a pain in her shoulders and upper back. During the steroid period, she hadn't once asked me to massage her back. *But one day in March, she did.* And she began to complain of bone pains, also for the first time in weeks. I knew what this meant. And I always had the impression that when things finally turned south again, they could move very quickly. *When you keep something going artificially for an extended period of time, you are only delaying the inevitable. Eventually the bubble will burst. And the more pressure you build up, the louder the pop.*

I had braced myself for this. Nadia, of course, avoided discussing it, at least with me. But at some point she would have no choice. Her condition began to deteriorate quickly, and the charade was coming to an end.

The Last Hurrah

With my realization that time was running out, I wanted to make sure Nadia enjoyed every minute she still had on this earth, with her friends, her husband, and especially her children. We had survived yet another brutal New York winter, and we were all desperate to get out of the house. The boys had a school break at the end of the month, and I had been contemplating what to do with that time.

One afternoon Nadia was lying in bed, and she called me over. I sat next to her and she held my hand. Nadia was, of course, aware of the upcoming school break and must have been thinking how best to utilize this precious time with her boys.

"Papa. Can I ask you something?"

"Of course, anything. What do you need? Are you hungry?" I replied.

She clinched my hand harder, and tears began to roll down her cheeks. In one of those rare windows when Nadia would choose to accept her condition—to acknowledge her reality—and in one of those moments that will remain engraved in my memory forever, she looked up at me and spoke through her tears.

"Papa. I want to see my boys' toes in the sand one last time."

She started sobbing and shaking. I burst into tears and clasped her hand as hard as I could. I couldn't contain myself. I couldn't be the strong one, not this time. The heartbreak of seeing her acknowledging her own imminent demise. The sadness and desperation in her eyes, quivering, knowing she would soon leave her boys. There wasn't a wish in the world I would not have killed to fulfill at that moment. We sat together, crying, sobbing, desperately holding each other. Until eventually, I caught my breath.

"Of course, Mama. Don't worry."

I left the room soaked in sweat and tears, hers and mine. She had asked for one last wish. And I was going to fulfill it.

I began thinking of what to do and where to go, and after a couple of days, I came up with a plan. The boys had really enjoyed a prior trip to the Bahamas, and I knew how much they loved the Caribbean. But this time we decided to go to the Cayman Islands instead. One of my dearest friends had retired there, and I thought a new destination would be fun for all of us.

Of course, this time around, Nadia was in no condition to handle commercial travel. She didn't have the energy to deal with the security lines and inevitable delays associated with commercial airlines. She also had to avoid crowded spaces, given her weak immune system (she had recently needed to leave a school play because the auditorium was being refurbished and the new "cafe-gymna-torium" had become too crowded). I knew how important this family time was, but getting her there as safely and comfortably as possible was also critical. So it would have to be different this time around.

One of Nadia's dreams had always been to travel on a private jet. I had done it a couple of times with an old friend, a retired ex-client, but I had never reserved one myself. So I called my friend, got the contact details of the lady who regularly arranged his flights, and set out to book our plane. It was, of course, a little extravagant for mere mortals such as ourselves, but this was no time to cut corners. I booked a Challenger 300 that comfortably seated nine people, in case Nadia wanted to invite her cousins or a couple of friends, which she did. I booked us at the Ritz-Carlton in Grand Cayman and even secured a beach cabana for the whole week. Nadia would have been too uncomfortable in the sun, and I didn't want her sitting in a room while her children were enjoying the beach. Suspecting this could be her last family holiday, I wanted it to be the trip of her life.

Nadia invited two of her cousins from Toronto and one of her dearest friends from Bronxville to come with us. They took turns taking care of her throughout the trip and managed to distract her and make her laugh. It made Nadia so happy to have them there with her, and I am grateful to them to this day for joining us on that trip. Yet despite the comfort of family and friends and the paradise-like setting, Nadia would not be able to escape her reality. During our time in Cayman I could see her getting increasingly tired and her cough worsening by the day. She attributed it mostly to the change of weather and air, having gone from the cold of New York to the hot, humid climate of the islands. This may have aggravated the cough somewhat, but I knew it wasn't the source.

While at the hotel, I was able to secure a wheelchair to move her around the resort's fairly vast grounds. Despite Nadia's weakening condition, we all managed to have a wonderful time. She was enjoying and appreciating every minute with an intensity I had never seen before. And although she never discussed it again, I could sense she knew this would be her final family holiday.

In retrospect, I know that had we planned the trip for just one week later, she wouldn't have been able to make it. *Somebody up above was looking after us. At least, it felt that way.*

Meltdown

Upon our return to New York, Nadia's condition declined precipitously. It was as if she had invested so much energy to make that final push (to make the trip, the last hurrah), that when she returned, her body just released. Her cough was taking on a whole new octave, and she was hardly able to make it up a flight of stairs. About three days later, she could barely walk. We had no choice but to call her doctors, who upon hearing her symptoms instructed me to take her to the clinic immediately.

When we arrived, the nurses (all dear friends of Nadia's by now) checked her vitals and went through the usual protocol. The doctor on duty ordered a CT scan to have a closer look at her chest, given that she was feeling weak and out of breath. This was her first scan in five months, and I was glad they were finally doing one.

Bizarrely, the scan showed some improvement in terms of the tumors in her lungs when compared to the previous scan. Normally, this would of course be wonderful news. Yet from a clinical

standpoint, her condition did not suggest any progress. Quite the contrary, she was visibly a lot worse.

One of the nurses, a very nice African American
woman who seemed to adore Nadia, did not appear
to agree with my assessment. "Nadia, you look
great, honey," she enthused as she took Nadia's
vitals. "What's happening? The scan was fine.
You're probably just tired from the trip. Maybe the
change of temperatures is affecting you."

This, of course, didn't make any sense. Nadia
had not exerted herself at all on that trip. One of the
reasons we took the jet was to ensure that would
be the case. There was no security line, there were
no crowds. They didn't even check our passports.
We basically walked into a small terminal where a
gentleman took our bags, and when the bags were
loaded onto the plane, Nadia was wheeled to the
aircraft. It took five minutes. The flight itself was
effortless. In fact, I would say it was relaxing. I
made sure our plane had a sofa so Nadia could take
a nap. And she did, on both legs of the flight. And
while at the hotel, she was wheeled everywhere and
took plenty of naps, in the room and the cabanas.

I knew something was wrong, and I was surprised the nurses were so nonchalant. Fortunately,
the doctor on call was actually willing to listen

more carefully. And was even willing to listen *to me*. But first I had to deal with the nurse.

"Yes, she may look better to you now. But we used a wheelchair to get her into the building. You only see her sitting down. I'm with her 24/7, and I don't think she is doing very well. She gets tired walking ten feet."

When the doctor came in to see us, she started asking all the right questions, the ones the nurses had seemed to brush aside. And when I explained to the doctor that Nadia's shortness of breath was getting bad, and that she was weaker by the day, the doctor paid attention. As I've mentioned before, there appeared to be an unwritten rule at Sloan Kettering whereby the staff would listen only to the patient, never the spouse. Again, I thought this was a mistake. *If you have a patient like Nadia, who wants to convince herself that everything is fine, she will never answer questions correctly. She will sugarcoat her answers to make herself believe what she wants to believe. Even worse, she will manipulate people around her into saying something that validates her own delusion.* The conversations that day were a perfect example.

"The cough has always been there. I just get tired, but it's probably just from the trip," Nadia said.

"Of course, because you look great. And maybe the change of air is affecting you. It could be anything. You look fine," replied the nurse.

I had been trained to bite my tongue in these situations. But everything has a limit. When the doctor finally came in, things changed. She was a youngish Irish woman who took the time to listen—to the patient and, uncharacteristically, *also the spouse.*

So I asked her, *"Doctor, I don't understand why there's such a contradiction between the scan, which looks a little better, and her clinical condition, which is decidedly worse?"*

The nurses had used a monitor to measure Nadia's oxygen intake. She was in the low 90 percents as she sat speaking with the staff. But on the basis of my insistence, the doctor conducted a little experiment. We would make Nadia walk down the hall and see what the intake would be when she was actually moving around. *It dropped to 80.* And that was the beginning of the downfall. The doctor made it clear she could not return home until her oxygen level improved, or until we had an oxygen system installed in the house. She would be hospitalized for three days to conduct tests and try to stabilize her breathing.

The H-Word

Up to that point, nobody had ever used the H-word (hospice). We knew that Nadia's condition was terminal, and that it was only a matter of time. But up to that point, the doctors had avoided using that term. In April 2015, that changed dramatically. *From that point on, the H-word was pretty much all we heard.* We were assigned a hospice nurse and social worker and were officially brought on board to the hospice services of Lawrence Hospital, run by a group called Jansen. We chose them because they had a good reputation and the hospital was near our house and the kids' school. We would bring Nadia home for as many days as possible under the care of our nurse, and she would be kept on oxygen from that point on. Despite the grim circumstances, Nadia was glad to be home. It was more comfortable and less stressful than being in a clinic, and most importantly, she was able to see her boys in a "normal" environment. During the home-hospice days, I believe Nadia truly understood the end was nearing. It was a huge relief for me to see that finally, after so many months of avoiding the obvious, Nadia was coming to peace with her impending fate. She seemed more introspective than ever. She told me how much she loved me over and over, and how grateful she was to have had the life she had and the husband she had. Hearing these words meant so much to me.

I had worked tirelessly throughout her illness to do absolutely everything I could to help her. During those long months, I never felt she appreciated any of it. This was made all the worse by her steroid outbursts. But somehow, during the hospice period, she changed. I derived a great deal of solace from that. I felt like for the first time, my dedication was acknowledged and appreciated. And in a much broader sense, I felt vindicated as a husband and as a man. I had always tried to give Nadia the best possible life I could. I was no rock star, but I worked extremely hard to give her as many earthly indulgences and experiences as I could, and to make her feel loved, safe, and free. To hear these words from her in those final days made me feel like all of my efforts, my work, my whole life—had been worthwhile.

The hospice days were also surreal in many ways. Despite knowing for months that this was where we were headed, that hospice care was inevitable—it still felt like a *shock*. The day Nadia's oncologist called to tell me that they could no longer treat her, and that hospice care was the next step, I almost fainted. *It made no sense. I had known this all along.* But sometimes you need to hear something from someone else for it to become real. My heart started pounding in my chest, and my legs felt like spaghetti. I was standing in my kitchen and almost fell over. I started hyperventilating and had to struggle to catch my breath. I was alone in the house at the time, so when I finally got ahold of myself, I started talking to myself to help process what was happening. "It's okay. It's okay. This was going to happen. It's okay. She won't suffer. Calm down. It's okay."

I managed to breathe into a rhythm and eventually got my bearings back. But I was shocked at just how *shocked* I was. I had always been told that nothing prepares you for moments like these. I now began to see how true this was. *And sadly, not for the last time.*

Grand Central Station

If the days between December and March had been hectic, the "headless chicken" phase, the hospice days were outright nuts. The flow of people coming in and out of the house was ridiculous. We had our nurse, Caroline, who came every day; her boss, the head nurse, who came every other day;

the social worker from Jansen also came every other day; and even our oncologist would stop by from time to time. We also had our nanny/home-worker, Kathy, who came three times a week, and a more comprehensive house cleaner, Marina, who came every Friday. And then there were relatives. My brother came over from Houston to provide me some much-needed support (this was a real blessing for me). Nadia's mother came over all the way from Dhaka, Bangladesh. One of her cousins from Toronto also came. And then there were the endless hordes of friends who came from all parts of the world to visit. Her friends from Bronxville and other parts of New York, of course, came by regularly. But we even had friends from Hong Kong, Madrid, and Miami make the trip. My house had become Grand Central Station!

All the while, there were day-to-day matters to attend to. There were forms to fill out and calls to make relating to Nadia's situation, as well as all of the boys' school and other activities, which required monitoring, and daily shopping, and plenty of other normal errands to run. The word "exhausting" does not begin to cover it.

Nadia and I were more than appreciative for all the love and kindness our friends and family demonstrated during those difficult days. I had a great relationship with pretty much all of them, and I loved the fact that they cared so much for her. But the traffic level during those hospice days was simply overwhelming. I was answering dozens of texts, fielding countless phone calls, and answering the door Lord knows how many times a day. It was all well-intentioned, I knew that. But it became too much for me, and more importantly, it became too much for Nadia.

At this stage Nadia was extremely weak. It was imperative for her to save her energy, especially for her children. Having friends over was nice, but it sapped a lot of energy from her, even if she wasn't the one doing the talking. One day it simply became too much. She had too many visitors and hadn't gotten enough sleep during the day. That night was hell, for her and for me. She was very short of breath all night, which triggered her violent coughing fits, which in turn fed the shortness of breath. I spent the night going back and forth regulating the oxygen levels to be sure she made it through each coughing fit. After that, we made it a point to regulate the visits. Without being disrespectful in any way to her many wonderful friends, we needed to limit the amount and length of the visits. The stakes were just too high.

Sister Morphine

We had managed to keep Nadia home on oxygen for three days at this point. But on the fourth day, I could see that she was visibly deteriorating. Her cough was intensifying, and now even speaking was an effort. So much so that she started writing on a little notepad to tell us what she wanted. She was too weak to really press down on the pen, so her lines were thin and sometimes difficult to read. She would also use her hands to make gestures and signs as a way of communicating with us. Her chest was so wrought with the disease, it was harder for her to speak than to move her arms. It was the most devastating thing in the world to witness. I had never really understood the technical definition of the word "invalid," but by all accounts, my wife of twenty years, my life partner, and the mother of my children had become one.

The decision to keep her at home or send her to inpatient hospice was becoming more pressing with each passing day. The hospice staff began to administer small doses of morphine to help ease the pain and discomfort. Our nurse, who did an amazing job throughout, managed to make it a lighthearted affair, convincing Nadia that taking morphine was no big deal, and that it was something that would help. Taking morphine, of course, has all sorts of stigmas associated with it, understandably. It is almost synonymous with end-of-life care. But it really helped with the pain, and we were fortunate to have access to it. My priority was that Nadia not suffer during her last days. And thanks to Nurse Caroline and her Sister Morphine, that was possible.

The Proudest Father

In mid-April, and bang in the middle of Nadia's home-hospice days, my older son, Ivan, got sick. We brought him home from school midday, and he was sporting a pretty high fever. We kept him on Tylenol until the next morning, when I could take him to a clinic to get checked out. While the two of us were alone in an exam room, waiting for the doctor to arrive, he looked down, rolling his fingers on the arm of his chair, and said, "Papa, how much longer do you think Mama has left?"

My heart raced as I tried to think of the best way to respond. But I was so happy that he was willing to have the conversation, as hard as it was. *That it came from him.*

"I don't know, son, but she's not doing very well at all."

"Do you think a year?"

"No, son, not a year."

"Do you think a month?"

"I'm not sure," I replied. "But definitely closer to a month than a year."

What he said next brought me to tears. I had to contain them because I knew the doctor was about to enter the room. But by the kindness of God, the doctor didn't come in, and Ivan was able to finish his thoughts.

"I think Mama will be much happier up there. I don't want her to bounce back only to go through all of this again. I don't want her to suffer anymore. It will be better when she is up there. She won't suffer there. It's just better."

I don't think it is possible to describe in words everything I felt at that moment—the sense of relief, and the overwhelming sense of pride as a father.

One of my biggest concerns had always been how my children would accept their mother's death. It was an issue that plagued me, something that kept me up most nights. We had *dealt* with the issue in some respects, a conversation here or there. But I had never really had my pulse on what was going on in their minds.

That day I understood where Ivan's head was. He had accepted his mother's imminent death, and he viewed it as positive relative to where she currently was. His sense of compassion for his mother's suffering outweighed his naturally selfish desire to keep her on earth, with him. It demonstrated a maturity and empathy I know I would have never had at just thirteen years of age. It also told me that despite his rather agnostic upbringing, he had developed Mommy and Daddy's sense of spirituality: a belief that there is something beyond this world, and that whatever that something is, it is good and peaceful.

I can say without reservation that it was the proudest day of my life as a father. In addition to the sense of relief I felt, knowing Ivan had come to terms with his mother's situation, I also saw his strength and his sense of humanity. And I knew that if he felt this way, it would make his little brother's grieving process all the easier. As with most siblings, Luca worshiped his older brother. If Ivan said Mommy was going to a better place, Luca would believe it. I told Ivan as we were getting into the car that day that I had never been more proud of him. *And as you read these lines now, my son, you should know how proud I am of you still.*

Window Pains

After a few days of home hospice, the bubble burst. It was all just too much. Nadia's condition had deteriorated, and her being home was doing more harm than good. When she was in the hospital just a few days prior, her oncologist had wanted her to go straight to inpatient hospice. But the on-call doctor had believed we had little to lose by trying to bring her home, at least for a couple of days (if that's what she wanted, of course). Nadia chose to try home care, understandably. But things at home deteriorated quickly.

I had a decision to make, one of the biggest of my life. I was Nadia's healthcare proxy, so I was pretty much in charge the second she could no longer make decisions for herself. In truth, we didn't need a legal document. Nadia had always relied on me to make decisions. She had a tendency to doubt herself when it came to big decisions, and she had always found security in my ability to be resolute, whether I was wrong or right. Sometimes I think it wasn't the actual logic behind my decisions that brought her a sense of security, but rather the conviction I conveyed in making them. I knew I could be wrong, but I was never afraid to commit.

So here we were. My son had just told me he could no longer bear to see his mother suffer, and yet there she was—ever weaker, ever closer to death, and ever more difficult to watch. The room she lay in, which had always been a place of warmth and security for the kids, where we had spent so many nights together watching TV, was now a place they dreaded to enter. *I knew that Nadia preferred being at home, but there comes a point where respecting someone's wishes begins to harm others. And as much as I loved her, I could not let that happen. I couldn't let the boys suffer any more than they already had.*

So that evening, I made the difficult decision that Nadia would be transferred to inpatient hospice. I spoke to our nurses and asked them to make the necessary arrangements. The next day, on April 17, Nadia left her home, never to return.

Death

On April 19, 2015, at 5:55 p.m., Nadia, my wife of twenty years, my life partner, and the mother of my children, passed away.

My memory of that day is not entirely clear, perhaps because of the frantic sequence of events, or maybe because my mind wants to block it out. But from what I do recall, Nadia did not suffer. She went peacefully, and I am grateful to the doctors who ensured that was the case.

For over an hour after she passed, I sat alone in that room, crying uncontrollably and telling her how much I loved her. I made the irreversible mistake of looking up and seeing her face and the whites of her eyes. I shouldn't have. That image kept me up for nights after, and it plagues me still. I pray that with the passage of time that image will be replaced with the memory of the beautiful, stunning woman I married. But for now, it haunts me. It is the picture of what death does. It takes. It takes everything. There was my Nadia, but my Nadia wasn't there. She was gone. There was nothing.

Death is nothingness. Death is ruthless, uncompromising, and merciless. It has no respect for time, place, or protocol. It cuts through everything. It takes no prisoners. It is absolute. I am not surprised that so many young soldiers return from war traumatized. Because seeing death up close changes you, forever.

Telling the Boys

When I left the hospital that night and returned home, I was paralyzed with fear about how I was going to tell my children that their mother had passed away. I knew this day was coming, and my boys of course sensed that their mother's end was near. But how do you actually tell them? I can say without reservation that the night of April 19, 2015, was the longest of my life. By the time I got home I was completely drained, physically and emotionally. I knew I did not have the strength to tell them that evening, and I didn't want them to deal with digesting the news overnight. So I decided I would wait until the next morning. It was a Sunday night, so I told the boys to go to bed because they had school the next day. Although I knew full well that they would not be going to school on Monday.

I spent the night agonizing about how to phrase something as horrific as their mother's death. I knew my words would mark them for the rest of their lives. It would be a moment that would torment them forever. How on earth would I tell them? I spent the night tossing and turning and petrified of the sunrise. But inevitably the time came.

The next morning, I walked up to the boys' room and told them softly to wake up. I stroked their hair and gave each of them a kiss. I was shaking. And in a trembling voice I told them.

"Ivan, Luca, Mama is finally resting. She is not suffering anymore."

The next few minutes scarred me for life and are engraved in my memory. They both burst into tears, Ivan silently, and Luca howling to the point of losing his breath. I tried to hold them and comfort them, telling them that it was okay, that their mother was safe now. But there was no stopping this. Luca repeatedly howled, "Why?" "Why?" They must have cried for an hour before gathering themselves.

I told them to stay home and that they didn't need to think about school for as long as they wanted.

We spent the rest of the day at home. And a quiet sadness filled the air of our silent house. A quiet sadness that would never leave us and one that we would have to learn to live with for the rest of our lives.

Ivan and Luca

To my spectacular sons, Ivan and Luca: this was the story of the final weeks and months of your mother's life. I don't know at what age you will read these lines, but I want you both to know that you were the most wonderful thing that ever happened to her. You filled her life with a joy beyond anything else in the world. And she was so proud of the young men you became. She will be looking down from above and continue to be proud of the two young gentlemen she raised. And Mama will never really be gone. She will always live in our hearts, and she will always live on through the two of you.

I don't know how well I was able to manage the circumstances. But I promise you both that I tried everything in my power to make those last weeks and months as bearable as possible for your mother. She fought bravely until the last minute. Not because she was afraid of dying, but because she wanted as much time as possible with the two of you, her treasures, her joy.

Ultimately, there was only so much I could do. Like the manager in a boxer's corner, I could provide screams of support and stand by her side. But there was only one boxer in the ring to fight the fight, and only she could win it. Ultimately, she did not.

And so your mother is no longer in this world. But your father is. And he will always be here for you. To love you and support you in all of your future endeavors. You are the pride and joy of my life, as you were your mother's.

I dedicate this book, as I do my life, to the two of you.

EPILOGUE

Life

As I write these lines, I have no idea what will become of my life. I don't know how long we will stay in Bronxville. I don't know what I will do professionally, or what will become of my life emotionally. Nadia would occasionally ask me, half-jokingly and half-seriously, to never remarry. She said I was hers and hers alone and that nobody else could have me. We would both laugh when she would talk this way. And I always joked back at her, telling her that this was the easiest promise in the world to keep!

But humor aside, I know what marriage entails. And I know what loving entails, at least for me. The experience I was forced to live through taught me much about the weight and responsibility of loving (again, at least for me). I have never known how to do things in half measures. My family and friends have always teased me about this. If I love, I love. And I do so unconditionally and without reservation. I would have happily exchanged my life for Nadia's at any point throughout her ordeal, without batting an eyelid. And I often thought about these sorts of things privately. The fact is that loving makes you vulnerable, and I am more aware of this today than I've been at any other point in my life. So I am naturally reluctant to even imagine myself ever loving or marrying another woman. But then again, what this experience also taught me is that you never really know what life is going to throw your way. I always loved the expression *"If you want to make God laugh, tell him your plans."* I finally understand it.

My priority now is to give my sons the best possible life I can. And to continue to embrace life with the same attitude I have always had. I have always viewed life as a gift worth treasuring every minute of every day, something I understand all the better now. I have never cared much about money or material things. They are only as good as the *fun* they can provide me or the experiences they can bring me. I have tried to instill in my children this philosophy as well. They should try to have fun no matter what they do, because life is a gift. Even when it comes to schoolwork, sports, or hobbies, I always told them they would never be any good at something they didn't enjoy. Figure out what you love and do *that*. The rest will fall into place.

I think this is one of the things Nadia liked most about me. I saw the positive in things and never let small things bring me down. I tried to stay at fifty thousand feet. It was better to be pound-wise, penny-stupid than the other way around. I was excited about seeing new places and doing new things. I've always had an appetite for the new and loved showing the boys all sorts of cool stuff.

At a deeper level, I have always believed life is nothing more than what you live and experience. I want to make sure that when I take my last breath, I can look back on a rich, action-packed life, full of all types of experiences, and with no regrets or unrealized dreams. It is *the moment and the experience* that matters. Because that is something nobody can ever take away from you. It isn't something you owned, it's something you *lived*. I would often joke with my friends that when we all get to the finish line, who really wins the race—the guy who has more money or the guy who had more fun? There was never a question in my mind. Not to say money is not important. We all need it to do the things we enjoy and to protect our families. But it isn't the priority. It's a means to an end, not an end in itself. If I got to the finish line and scored highest in the "fun per day" or "laughs per hour" categories, I would consider myself the winner.

I know I will always carry the scar of losing my wife. I know I will be forever changed by it. But I will not let it change my DNA. There are plenty of *moments* ahead. And I plan on making as many of them as I can.

What If?

As I reflect on Nadia's illness and death, I can't help but ask a few what-ifs. It is clear that the single most important weapon we have against cancer is early detection. Nadia had her breasts checked every year—but skipped one. Fatefully, it was the year she developed the disease. By the time we began to treat it, it was already too late. The five positive lymph nodes told us as much. But what if she had been checked that year? Would we have caught it in time? Would we have stopped it before it spread to her lymphatic system?

And what about some of the decisions made in her treatment? Our first surgeon at Lawrence advocated neoadjuvant therapy, whereby chemo is administered first, to see if the tumors react to the treatment. The surgery itself (the mastectomy) is conducted afterward, once the doctors are confident they have the most effective chemo agents to combat the disease. But the second surgeon, whom we would eventually stick with (at Weill Cornell), advocated traditional adjuvant treatment, whereby the breast is removed first and the chemo is administered afterward. We decided on the second surgeon on the basis that she was more experienced and was considered a sort of celebrity in her field. *In retrospect, that may have been a mistake.* After Nadia's cancer recurred, I asked our oncologist how the cancer could have returned so quickly. Her response: *It was the wrong chemotherapy.*

So maybe the neoadjuvant approach would have made more sense. What if we had tested the first chemo regimen (AC-T) on the tumor and saw there was no reaction? Then we could have tried other agents until we found one that worked. With the traditional adjuvant treatment, we never had that option.

And then there is the what-if related to the testing of the all-important hormone receptors. Nadia was initially diagnosed as triple negative using a test called IHC (immunohistochemistry). About a year later, after Nadia had finished her chemotherapy, her oncologist decided to test again using a different method, called fluorescence in situ hybridization (FISH). The FISH test is used less often, because it is more complicated and more costly. But it is known to be more accurate. When the FISH method was finally used, she actually expressed slightly for HER2 and ER. This means that we could have used some targeted hormone therapies in parallel to the chemo all along. But we didn't, because we only used the IHC test at initial diagnosis, which didn't pick up on the HER2 and ER expressions later detected by the FISH test. What if the FISH test had been run from the beginning? Would they have been able to use a targeted hormone treatment in addition to the chemo? Would it have worked?

All in all, I can say we were privileged to have access to the medical resources we had. The doctors were excellent, and the level of service throughout was exceptional. But without being a doctor myself, I am still left with some questions. *What if?*

ACKNOWLEDGMENTS

There are a number of people I would like to recognize and thank for making this book possible. I would like to firstly thank my many friends around the world for all of their love and support during the very difficult period when these pages were written. You are far too many to mention individually, but you were all an indispensable source of strength to me. A special word of thanks to Sherry Lawrence in Los Angeles for convincing me that my story was one worth sharing, and one that may help others get through the agonizing and lonely task of trying to save a loved one. Thank you to the exceptional team of professionals at Girl Friday Productions in Seattle for their belief in my message and for their extraordinary patience throughout this process. And finally, a very special word of thank you to my brother, Carlos, without whom I would have never survived this ordeal, or any other, for that matter. You are and have always been the most important constant in my life. *Te quiero.*

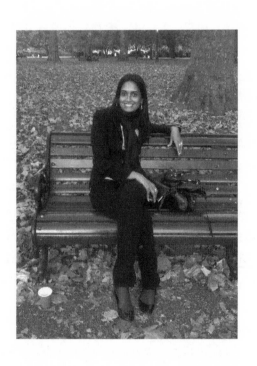

ABOUT THE AUTHOR

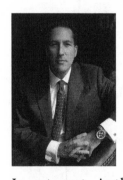 Miguel Barron, CFA, is a retired investment banker living in Los Angeles with his two sons, having retired following the passing of his late wife. He began his career in 1992 as an investment analyst at the Abu Dhabi Investment Authority, based in Abu Dhabi. In 1995 Barron moved to London and later New York, where he would work on the international equity desks of prominent investment banks, including Santander, Robert Fleming, BT Alex Brown, and most recently UBS. A graduate of the University of California at Santa Barbara, Barron holds a master's degree in international economics from the Johns Hopkins School of Advanced International Studies. He has been a CFA charter holder since 2001. Barron is the founder and managing partner of US Traveler Assist, a global network of former senior US Embassy officials assisting US travelers abroad. *The Boxer's Corner* is Barron's first book.

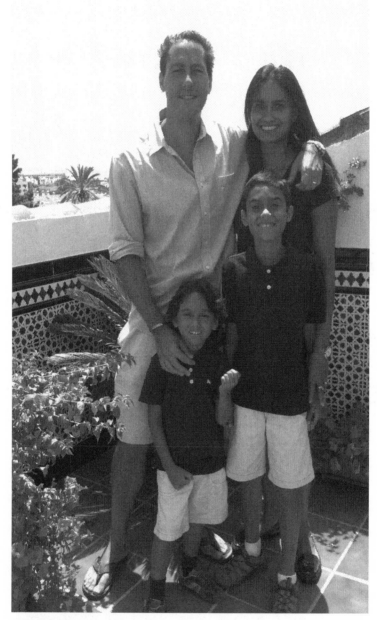

Marbella, 2011

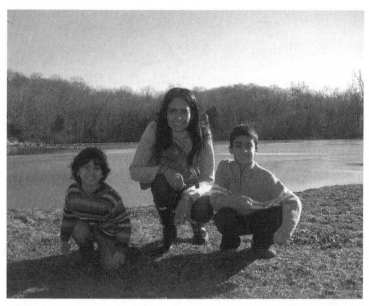

Pennsylvania, 2008

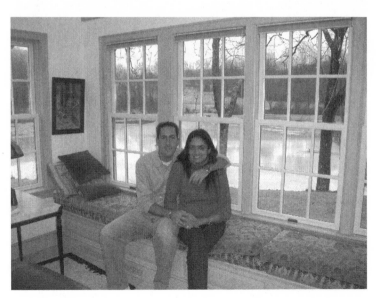

Pennsylvania, 2008

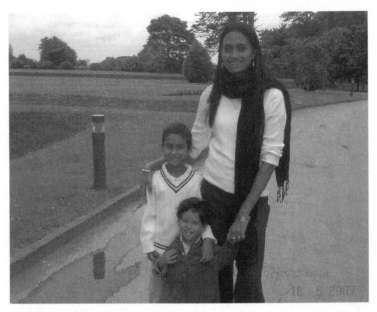

Ireland, 2007

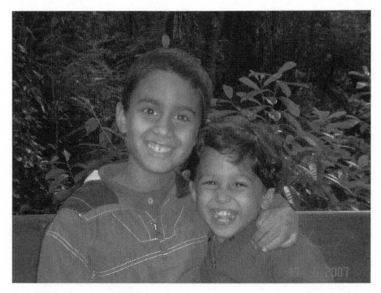

Ireland, 2007

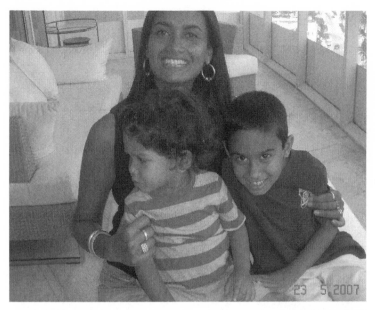

South Beach, 2007

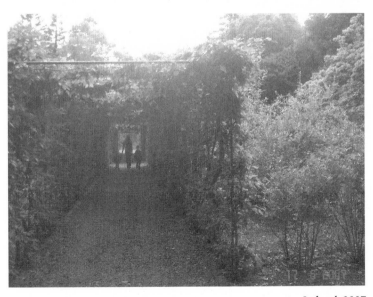

Ireland, 2007

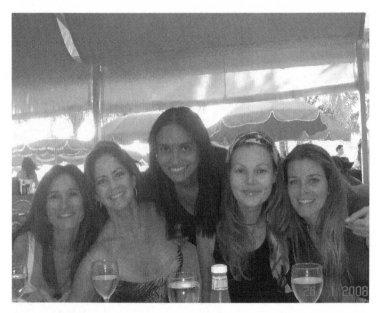

Miami, 2008

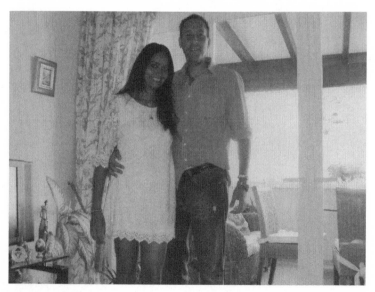

Marbella, 2010

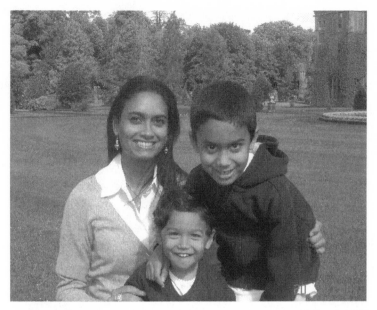

Ireland, 2007

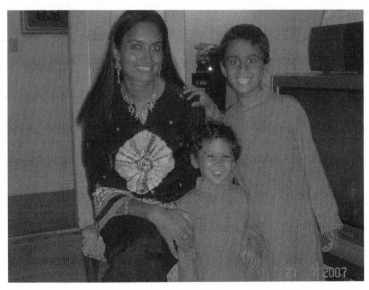

Toronto, 2007

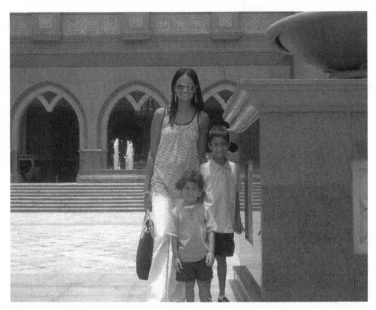

Abu Dhabi, 2008

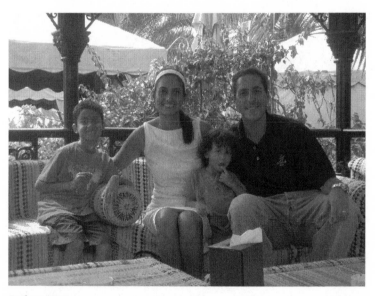

Dubai, 2008

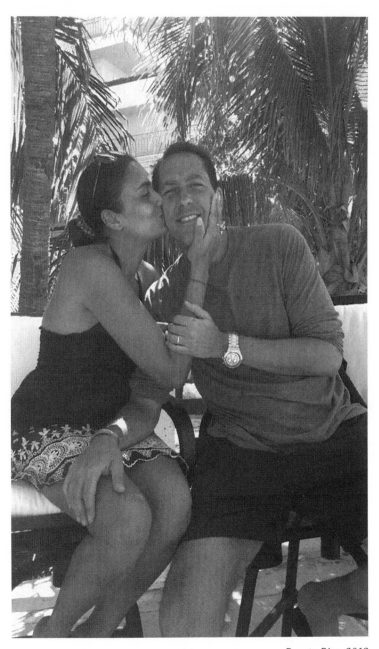

Puerto Rico, 2012

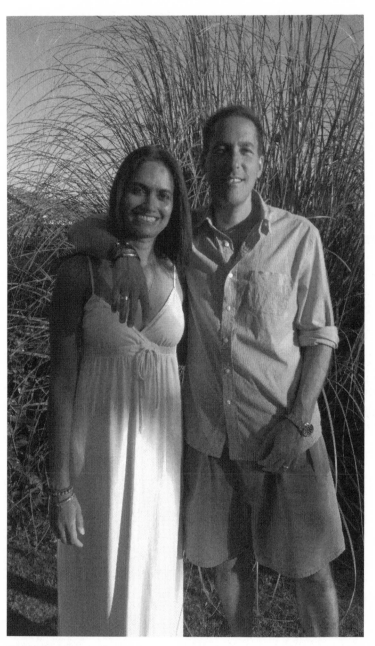

Marbella, 2012

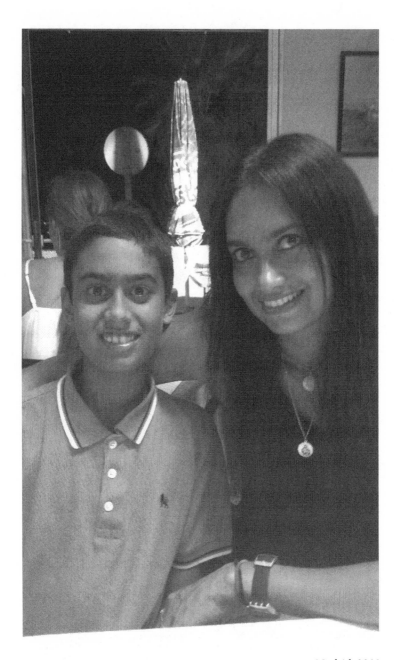

Madrid, 2011

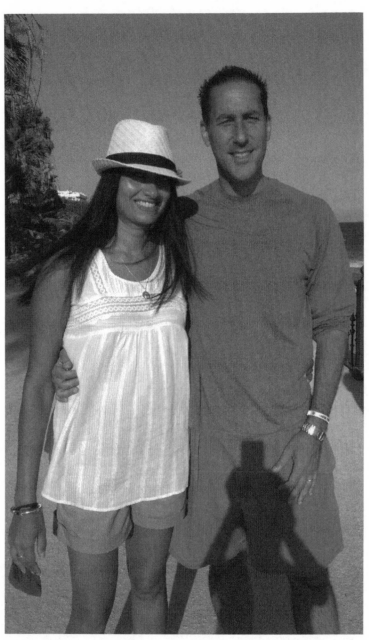

Marbella, 2010

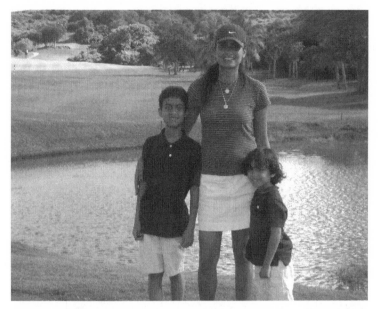

Doral, 2006

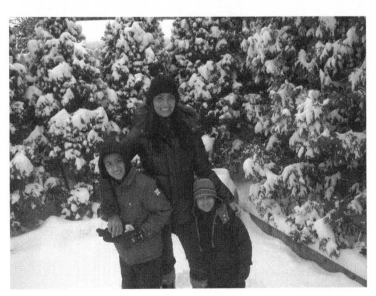

Bronxville, 2010

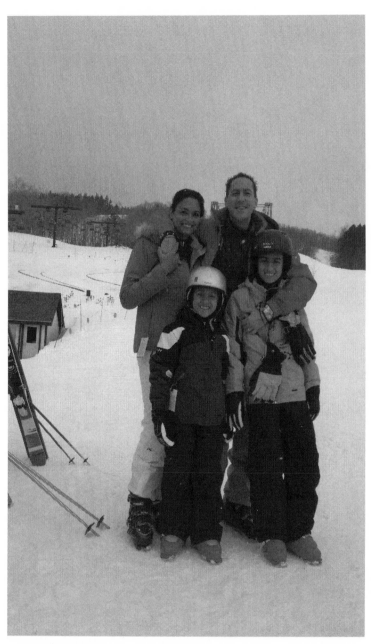

Beaver Creek, 2013

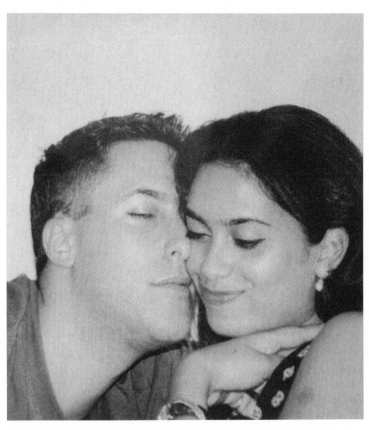

Our first picture together, Abu Dhabi, 1995

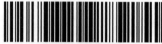
42638299R00092

Made in the USA
Lexington, KY
18 June 2019